THE

RedWine

DIET

ENJOY LIFE.
LOSE FAT.

ART MCDERMOTT

CSCS CISSN

Book design & eBook conversion by manuscript2ebook.com

About the Author

Art McDermott
Owner – Wellness Consulting Group
Co-Founder & COO National Corporate Fitness Institute

Art McDermott CSCS CISSN is a Certified Nutritionist and has been a Certified Strength and Conditioning Specialist for 30 years.

Art has spent years in the corporate wellness arena; conducting speaking, corporate trainings, "boot camp" sessions as well as custom fitness programs. Art works with large and small businesses helping them deal with the issues surrounding an aging workforce as well as the productivity and success of executives and all members of the "road warrior" population.

In the private sector, he has owned several training facilities specializing in personal training, nutrition, fitness/physique transformations, 'baby boomer' and senior training as well as sports preparation. Art has been involved with strength sports for over 25 years. During that time, he has participated in over 20 National and World Championships in three different sports, in addition to 2 Olympic Track & Field Trials.

Current highlights:

- Author, Professional Speaker, Consultant and Wellness Activist

- Adjunct Professor – University of Massachusetts, Lowell. College of Health Sciences.

- 4 Time NCAA All-American in Track & Field and a member of multiple US National and International Teams

Art focuses the much of his time on the *"Boomer Blueprint"*; a product and service designed specifically for helping individuals 50 years of age and over retain or regain their health vitality and independence. Art is also known for his work helping personal trainers grow their businesses focusing on this older population.

Current Published Books:

"Boomer Blueprint – A Step-by-Step Guide to Longevity, Anti-Aging and Fitness for Baby Boomers"

"The Red Wine Diet – Enjoy Life. Lose Fat."

Please contact Art directly for details about having him speak to your group or organization.

"The Wine Guy" Contributor

Jeff Slavin

BA International Political Economy - Clark University 1983

M ED - Lesley University 1992

Jeff has over 20 years of experience in the fine wine business. He is currently the owner of Hangtime Wholesale Wine Company, selling artisan wine to the Massachusetts market.

Married to Lori, with a Step-Son Matt and a Puggle named Manny.

Hobbies: Jazz music and my 'Old Man Softball League'

Table of Contents

INTRODUCTION

Who is this book for?

This book is for anyone who is NOT interested in a 'diet'.

Yes, I used the word "diet" in the title, but besides showing you how to eat the right foods while not giving up your pinot, I present an actual lifestyle which will help you lose weight, keep it off for the long haul and help you live a longer more fulfilling life.

(NOTE: Throughout this book, I will most often refer to *"The Red Wine Diet"* as an "approach" rather than a diet. You will understand why soon enough...)

More importantly, this book is for people who need a simple yet realistic approach that they can actually stick with without feeling like they are living on salads and carrot sticks; and who want to enjoy an active life sharing fun times with friends and family.

This book is also written for anyone in their 40's, 50's, 60's and beyond who may have to re-learn almost everything they know about food. Why?

In no uncertain terms, you have been lied to. In fact, you have been lied to on a long-term and institutionally-accepted scale for a long, long time.

It is not the consumer's fault. Even those who teach us about health were taken in by the pervasive lies. I had a college professor during the 1980's who proudly displayed a cup with the statement "I never met a carbohydrate I didn't like." Clearly he was indoctrinated into the "low-fat, high carb" mentality which dominated the era. This is a professor of physiology, with access to all the latest facts and data, yet he was still convinced all carbohydrates were good and all fat was evil.

If a man of science within the realm of human physiology could be taken in, what chance did the average consumer have?

You don't have to be a nutritionist to lead a healthy lifestyle, but you do need to understand your food; its sources and its effects upon your health. The more education you gather, the more approaches like 'The Red Wine Diet' will make sense to you.

Imagine finding out most of the nutritional facts you learned growing up were wrong. Not just wrong, but these facts were intentionally manipulated, and then ingrained in American culture to the point of universal acceptance. Sounds outrageous doesn't it?

I am not a conspiracy theorist by any stretch. I don't think the government is listening to my conversations on my phone. If they were, they would be disappointed and bored very quickly...

However, as a result of poor science, manipulated government policy and shady industry ethics, Americans have been 'fed' decades of lies about our food supply and what is good for us. These myths are so pervasive in the American consciousness, when I mention them in presentations, people are shocked.

"What do you mean fat is not bad for us?"

"How can you say grains are not good for us?"

It goes on and on...

"I thought the FDA was supposed to be on our side. Why have I not heard this before? " they ask.

You will hear it now. As cynical as it sounds, in many cases it simply a matter of money. Many of the reasons factual information is not more readily available is largely because there is little profit to be made from a population eating plenty of fruits and vegetables, moderate dairy, moderate red meat.

"Free Range" is not a marketing term; it is how animals are supposed to be raised.

"Organic" is not a new approach; it is how everyone ate before food processing.

"Farm to Table" is not some novel concept; it is the way humans ate for hundreds and hundreds of years.

The word "diet" implies a short-term fix. Personally, I don't like the word. Wouldn't it be better to have a truly viable approach that you can sustain for a life-time? Diets don't work. Lifestyles work. Good long-term habits work. Quick fixes never work.

In this book, we will provide you with simple check lists and guidelines to follow. I'm a huge fan of the 'bullet point summary'. Information presented the way we think, and more importantly, in a way we will remember.

This book is for people looking to lose body fat, manage their weight, and to sustain a healthy lifestyle on a new set of terms.

You still want to enjoy life. You may also enjoy wine. You are hopefully willing to 'disrupt' the way you currently think about food, and re-structure a lifestyle assuring weight management and overall health.

Who is this book NOT for?

If you believe you may have an issue with alcohol, this book is not for you. I advocate reasonable and controlled amounts of wine. If you lack control when it comes to alcohol consumption, or have a history of alcoholism, please do not use this book as an excuse to imbibe to excess.

It must be stated; it is relatively easy to exceed the recommended amount of alcoholic drinks per week found in this book. There is an abundance of science showing the dangers of too much alcohol. Excess intake has been linked to breast cancer in women. Liver damage and impaired functioning are the better known consequences.

Use caution and moderation at all times. Finally, be honest with yourself. If you believe you have an issue, please seek qualified counseling. Of course, women who are pregnant should not consume alcohol.

INTRODUCTION

If you are looking for a weight loss quick fix, this may not be your ideal choice for a solution. This is not to say that by following this solution, the changes you will see in your body can't happen quickly. In fact, by removing the foods on our "Banned Foods List" you may feel better almost immediately. However, we will be emphasizing a long-term, lifestyle-based solution…again, not a 'diet'.

The Starting Point

When I sat down to write this book, I knew I did not want to write a workout book. There is an abundance of information across the internet and on every newsstand about how to work out, what exercises to do, how often, etc. I will admit, my colleagues and I are all about the hard workouts utilizing different workout structures, varying levels of intensity, and the latest program designs, all producing remarkable results. After all, this is what we have done for years.

If you are looking for appropriate, successful training programs, I have additional resources for you, designed specifically to show you what your workouts should look like "at our age". My first book, "Boomer Blueprint" goes into great detail about how to build a proper workout. I recommend you seek out this book if you want a great introduction to fitness training. You can find it at www.boomerblueprint.com.

You will also see some crossover of the themes in this book and the points introduced in the *"Boomer Blueprint"*. Why? Because these things work! Why change them…

While there is a place for properly designed fitness programs, it's not here. Here, I will tell you how to achieve significant results without hours in the gym, and especially without running mile after mile on the treadmill or on the road.

One thing all my fellow fitness colleagues agree upon is that nutrition accounts for 65-70% or more of your weight management results. Meaning, you could have the greatest workouts in the world, but still be a complete physical wreck without proper nutrition.

As the saying goes, "You cannot out-train a poor diet."

The point is, if you are looking for a challenging workout guide, this is not that book. Many people I spoke with while writing this book had very little interest in regular strength training at all. I get it. As much as I am an advocate of strength training, I am the first to admit weight loss is easily achieved without killing yourself in the gym.

INTRODUCTION

I have been a Certified Strength and Conditioning Specialist since the first certification exam was created by the National Strength & Conditioning Association in the mid 1980's. Even though I am a "fitness guy", and have been lifting weights for approximately 40 years, I chose a decidedly different direction by moving away from the 'fitness 'theme in writing the *"Red Wine Diet"*.

Again, what I really set out to define through *'The Red Wine Diet'* is more of an approach...not a diet...not a workout program...not deprivation regiment. This is simply a way to live day in and day out, in a manner which leads to more vibrant health, body fat loss and on-going weight management.

Once you have successfully achieved your desired weight by following the simple guidelines in this book and you see your health take a huge turn for the better; then maybe we can have a conversation about what should come next. However, let's take one thing at a time. For now, we will focus our efforts on The Red Wine Approach to weight loss. Lifting glasses and forks loaded with the right stuff in the right amounts is our goal.

We will tell you exactly what foods to increase or introduce into your daily routine. It seems every other week some new study comes out telling us a certain food – once thought to be evil – is now in favor. And vise versa, some food once thought to be the cornerstone of health is now killing us. We will clarify all the misinformation.

We will also weed out the foods which sabotage our efforts to maintain or lose weight over time. I can't pigeon-hole *"The Red Wine Diet"* into a convenient category such as "South Beach", "Mediterranean" or "Zone" etc. The components you see here come from all over and simply make sense.

What has been removed from *"The Red Wine Diet"* solution is a few decades of lies. We attack the status quo and get back to how you should be eating.

That being said, one of the primary contentions of this book is the "you can have your cake and eat it too" attitude. Yes, you can have your wine, eat some dessert and lose weight. It can be done.

You will learn the subtle changes you can make which will guide you away from that slow, steady and dangerous weight gain many of us experience as we age.

We will also show you how you can slowly modify your own behavior, so actions and decisions you once struggled with will now be under your control.

As a certified nutritionist, I have read the science and have studied a myriad of nutritional plans. I have helped clients lose literally thousands of pounds of body fat using a wide variety of plans. However, along the way, I noticed something. The people who took severe approaches to weight loss were no more successful over the long haul at maintaining a healthy body weight than anyone else. In addition, the people who savored life, ate good foods, and yes, drank a little wine saw more success, seemed happier along the journey, and kept the weight off longer.

There is not a 'one-size-fits-all' answer here.

However, there are common threads which appear in the approaches used by those who are successful at weight management, as well as happy and healthy. We will focus our attention there.

Now...let's address the big red elephant in the room. Can you really drink wine and lose weight? Absolutely! Alcohol intake and robust health need not be mutually exclusive, as long as certain recommendations are followed.

I enjoy wine, predominately red wine. I also have every intention of living a long, active and healthy life. I am striving to be "that guy" who can still handle long hikes on a trial somewhere when I am in my 70's and 80's and who has plenty of energy to spare. I want my stress to be at a minimum, and my enjoyment to be plentiful.

One thing I knew enough not to do was just "hope" for this long, healthy life, without having a plan to get there.

All too often many of us let life happen to us instead of being more actively and consciously involved with choosing our direction. I realized that if I did not stay on top of things I could find myself standing in my own way. When we neglect our health, we suddenly wake up and realize we can't live the life we wanted because our body and its complex systems have started to break down, much like any machine, when neglected.

I needed more structure than that...hence, the birth of *"The Red Wine Diet"*.

In keeping with my desire for simplicity and my background in teaching, I start each section of this book with a short list of "Objectives" and then proceed to explain each one in detail. At the end of each section, I list out for you important

INTRODUCTION

"Take Away Action Items".

This structure will go a long way towards helping you remember the key points being made, make them easier to come back to in the future, and provide simple action steps to assure your success.

Finally, I am very excited about the chapters on wine itself. Wine expert, Jeff Slavin has taken what can be a complex subject – wine tasting and selection – and created a straightforward guide for all of us. I sought out Jeff because I wanted to provide the same clarity to the subject of wine as I hope I have presented on the subject of food. Jeff has done that through his simple and open-minded approach to wine and wine selection.

- **Art McDermott**

As the years go by, and we look for ways to live right, eat better and maintain or improve a healthier lifestyle, knowing more about what we consume has never been more important. This book hopes to inform consumers of the overall health benefits of wine as a casual beverage in the context of a balanced approach to diet and exercise. We hope to provide a friendly and practical guide to some of the growing body of evidence of the positive health benefits found in wine. We will also try to guide you through the vast body of information on the world of wine, demystifying and simplifying a beverage that has been with us for thousands of years.

- **Jeff Slavin**

CHAPTER 1

Disruption & Mindset

"Where the mind goes, the man follows"
- Proverbs 23:7

Objectives:

1. To realize success (in just about anything) begins and ends with balance

2. To understand that in order to break a long-term habit, often significant disruption is necessary

3. To create realistic goals

4. To recognize and fight the "resignation mindset"

5. To see how Pareto's Rule applies to your world

When I wrote the *"Boomer Blueprint"*, a book that gets into strength training for people over age 50 in great detail, my co-author and I spent a great deal of time discussing 'mindset'.

As most of you know, unless you have complete mental "buy-in" to any program or diet, it is unlikely that you will succeed. This also easily applies to a relationship, a job, or any project you take on. However, if you are in the right mindset and can go all in, your chances of success are greatly enhanced.

The mind controls everything. The challenge comes with getting into and maintaining the right state of mind.

CHAPTER 1

Here are some recurring themes which, once engrained, should become your 'mantra for success'. While these themes may seem contradictory, they actually work powerfully together.

1. ***The Red Wine Diet* is all about disruption.** This theme is a powerful one, but all too often overlooked. The idea of disruption refers to the concept of breaking free from your rote behaviors and way of thinking, and plugging into something new. Most of us live our lives following deeply engrained comfort patterns without thinking of the benefits or consequences. We spend day after day simply going through mechanical acts such as eating, sleeping, commuting, and aging without any careful thought going into our decisions in these areas.

If your existing patterns have landed you in a poor situation, it often requires a disruption to bring about needed change.

On a small but personally important scale, here is one example from my life.

When I sold my fitness facility, I suddenly found myself without a workplace to travel to on a daily basis. My intent was to write, consult and produce fitness and wellness related content. I no longer had employees asking questions, or large numbers of clients seeking me out on a daily basis. Good, right?

Not necessarily. I also found myself without any true form of a daily schedule. My day revolved around when I would break for lunch or even snacks, and I even found my workout times drifting through various points of the day without any rhyme or reason.

I quickly realized that I preferred a bit more structure to my day. In order for me to be productive, I needed to disrupt the way I had now designed my day.

My solution was to change my workout time to the first thing in the morning; something I had never done in my 40 years of strength training. I started to get up at 5:30am to get my workout done. Guess what I discovered?

I had more energy throughout the day and had gained considerably more time, since I no longer had to plan for taking an hour or more later in the day for training. I was instantly more productive. I took an otherwise unused portion of my day and filled with a beneficial activity. (It didn't hurt when I read about many of the most successful people in the world starting off their day by working out first thing in the morning!)

CHAPTER 1

I was hooked. I now train regularly in the morning, having successfully disrupted a lifelong pattern and replaced it with a new and better one.

On a far larger scale, we can see positive disruptions all around us. In my opinion, some of the best examples of positive disruptions are Elon Musk and Uber.

As of this writing, Elon Musk is changing the auto industry with his Tesla brand electric cars. He is also looking to get every home in the country powered by electricity. In addition, he is the central figure in Space X; the first successful, privately funded "space transport" company. One might call him disruptive to say the least. He has taken the status quo and promptly ignored it.

And as of today, the ride hailing app Uber is fundamentally changing the taxi industry by circumventing the traditional 'ride for hire' services by using private drivers to lower fares. Many people who are against services like Uber find themselves trying to hold back the tide with a tablespoon. I equate these arguments to those who might lament to loss of the milkman coming to your door. While it may have had some advantages, it is simply an era long gone by.

The industry has been disrupted forever and will never be the same.

I consider Elon Musk and Uber to be elements of disruption. Each of us should create our own smaller version of these. I constantly encourage clients to honestly look for ways they can introduce similar disruptions into their own lives in order to evoke positive change.

Being open to this mindset is crucial. If you are determined to stick to your existing ways because these habits provide a level of comfort, you cannot be surprised when nothing changes. If you do what you have always done, you will get what you have always got.

Disruption is the only real way out; stepping out of you comfort zone, as the cliché goes.

Examples of small yet viable disruptions to evoke positive lifestyle changes include:

- Early morning workouts (or simply starting an activity such as regular walking)

- Earlier bedtime

- Replacing soda with water

- Dropping a food from your diet which may taste great, but is clearly a problem for you

- Taking up a new stress reduction activity such as yoga or meditation

- Replacing one indulgence with one which may lead to better habits, say replacing beer with wine or replacing ice cream with dark chocolate

- Consciously minimizing portion sizes; perhaps buy going out and buying smaller plates

- Scheduling in 'downtime' for yourself rather than falling into the go-go mentality, which is erroneously rewarded in our society today

- Scheduling fixed times to meet with friends and family, which may have been lost to our daily grind

Notice that these changes are not massive in scale. From my experience, people who try to make huge wholesale changes open themselves up to failure. Small realistic, incremental changes are best. They are easier to implement and easier to sustain. In addition, celebrating a series of small victories breeds long-term success!

It's OK to reward yourself when you have succeeded in making a positive change, no matter how small.

2. *"The Red Wine Diet"* **is all about balance.** Creating the ideal mindset to achieve weight loss involves much more than counting calories. You must strive to achieve balance with:

   O   Work with Family/Play time

   O   Sleep with Wakefulness

   O   Stress with Relaxation

   O   Training with Recovery

When all of these issues are in balance, weight management becomes easy. Much has been said and written about the "wine lifestyle". I leave the details about that to my far more oenophilic co-author, Jeff Slavin. I will say, however, that this lifestyle balance is far more about dedicating an evenly proportionate amount of time to more social activities and time spent focusing on the enjoyment of food, friends, and family. In short, this refers to non-stressful pursuits evoking balance and enjoyment. We will discuss the trauma brought on by stress in a coming section.

This theme of balance and enjoyment provides subtle, yet powerful benefits. The more you think about it, the more it becomes impossible not to see the parallel between the degradation of our food supply and the degeneration of our current lifestyles both brought on by 'progress'. Just as our food has seen a growing imbalance in the nutrients comprising it, our lives have seen an equally dangerous and negative imbalance between overwhelming stress and a healthy quality of life at a slower, more natural pace.

3. **The counter to making small successful changes is what I refer to this as the "Resignation Mindset".**

   The "Resignation Mindset" can be seen in that huge percentage of the population showing the following characteristics:

   – At least 20-30 pounds of excess body fat

   – Possess feelings of guilt, disappointment or angst about their excess body weight. They see someone in the mirror who they never planned on looking or feeling like.

- Possess feelings of guilt about the long-term failure to act upon something that they KNOW is a danger to their longevity

- Show a somewhat defeated 'resignation' about how they look and feel, as if it is almost too late to change the way they are.

- May suffer from a 'paralysis by analysis' regarding the steps necessary to make a change. They are overwhelmed by conflicting information in the media or just the sheer volume of information floating around the internet on the topic of weight loss, and *therefore do nothing.*

A significant part of the reason why many people find themselves in this situation stems from a point I raised in the Introduction. Much of the information about our food that those of us in the United States today have been taught is a complete lie.

By no means does this give everyone a free pass to treat their health as an afterthought. KNOWING you have been lied to provides you with a mandate to change.

CHAPTER 1

Where should you start?

Here is a list of habits or mindsets that can and will crush your dreams of robust health. These are items many do without forethought, but perhaps through resignation to their circumstances.

- Eating late-night, high-sugar foods

- Accepting a sedentary lifestyle

- Eating one giant meal in the evening and next to nothing the rest of the day

- Not being mindful of sugar and processed carbohydrate intake

- Not taking corrective measures against stress

- Not working up a sweat occasionally

- Accepting excess bodyweight as being inevitable

A Word About Goal Setting...
Finding Your 'Why'?

As I have mentioned, people who take a highly disciplined, even severe approach to weight loss often fail. Why is that? Why is it that many of us can start off with all the best intentions and still fail?

In the excellent book, "The Power of Full Engagement", authors Jim Loehr and Tony Schwartz suggest a remarkably simple explanation.

Self-discipline is an exhaustible resource.

If you are relying on a deep well of self-discipline to get you to your goal, you are faced with a high probability of failure. Your initial "iron will" fades with time. Old habits creep back in. It is our natural tendency to revert to old patterns because they are comfortable. When we do this, we quickly find ourselves facing the same vicious cycle of poor health, and the nagging guilt associated with it; the need to try another quick fix, another failure, etc.

Your goals and hence your 'new' mindset must be driven by a deeper emotional reason in order to sustain the fire towards success.

CHAPTER 1

Therefore, before you define your goals, before you lay out your new diet and before you buy that case of red wine, you must first determine the true emotional reasons why you need to make this change. There are as many possibilities for answers here as there are readers.

Are you motivated (or scared) by medical news? Have you been through a change in your relationships or have the desire to improve one? Have you suffered the loss of someone near to you, and seek to address your own longevity? Have you been through a recent divorce? Has stress taken over your life to such a degree that you realize stress reduction is no longer optional, but is necessary for your very survival?

It is up to you to have this deep and honest conversation with yourself to determine your answer. It is also imperative to remove any vagueness about your new mission.

This won't happen overnight. In fact, the science says if you can stay true to a new pattern or habit for a minimum of 21 days, your likelihood of success dramatically increases. Here is how that mindset shift works. Let's say your new habit is lifting weights at the gym 3 days per week... a noble goal. At first, it may feel a bit like drudgery, especially if lifting weights is fairly new to you, and you have yet to develop a feeling of comfort with the machines, your workouts, the locker rooms, etc.

However, with time, this discomfort will slowly disappear. *The gym magically transitions from something you **have** to do to something you simply '**do**'.* It becomes a regular part of your day. Something you schedule in without even thinking about it.

Those around you are now aware of your schedule, and accept it as part of your routine. This means you now have a tacit support system. You have introduced a valuable new habit which may very well stay with you for years and even decades.

That being said, let's talk about how to, stay 'compliant' to any new routine in the face of slip ups and challenges. Remember, once you have determined your goal and defined your emotional reasons for wanting to achieve this goal, compliance does indeed become easier.

First, don't be so hard on yourself. Everyone screws up. Overindulgence of sugar and/or alcohol happens to just about everyone. Everyone lapses. It's the length of the lapse which determines the impact. This means, as long as you get back to your healthy way of eating, working, etc. as quickly as possible, you will minimize the 'damage' caused by your brief lapse.

Unfortunately, when people screw up their health plan by making a poor decision, they often resign themselves to failure, and scrap their entire health planning for extended periods. They throw their hands up in the air and tell themselves they can't do it.

The upside to this is, *"The Red Wine Diet"* is not about harsh periods of denial. Once you understand the specific foods you need to avoid and slowly begin to follow a new pattern, staying on track becomes an afterthought.

Think of compliance this way. We are going to paraphrase the now-famous "Pareto Rule", otherwise known as the 80/20 rule. This rule was first proposed by Vilfredo Pareto, an Italian economist, and first put forward in 1896. The rule states that 80% of the effects come from 20% of the causes.

We will put a different twist on this very versatile rule.

"The Red Wine Diet" Rule:

80% of your weight loss results will come if you screw up no more than 20% of the time

Does this approach take a bit longer than some diets following more severe rules? Perhaps, but keep in mind, our goal is long-term lifestyle changes, not necessarily speed. With speed often comes failure and the tendency to regain weight. (If you are looking for techniques to speed up your results, check out *Chapter 7 – The Accelerators,* for additional options.)

When we slow down and weight loss becomes a steady process, compliance increases and our new habits become engrained for the long-term.

When you start to think of your health as a marathon and not a sprint, you start to understand the state of mind needed for success.

All of these factors contribute to a longer fuller life:

- More social activity = longer life

- Decreased sugar = longer life

- Stress reduction = longer life

- Less processed food = longer life

- Balance = longer life

CHAPTER 1

Action Item "Take-aways":

1. Identify the areas in your life where you believe you lack balance

2. Plan out a specific (preferably small) "disruption" to your daily routine, and execute this disruption for a minimum of 21 days while specifically addressing the above imbalance.

3. Follow Pareto's Rule for your health. Stay compliant 80% of the time and make your 'lapses' very brief.

"Only the wisest and stupidest of men never change"

- Confucius

CHAPTER 2

Is Red Wine REALLY Healthy?

– Jeff Slavin

Objectives:

1. To review a brief history of how wine came to be in the first place

2. To discuss the health effects most commonly associated with wine consumption

Wine as an everyday beverage has been with human civilization nearly since we crawled out of the caves. There is plenty of evidence of wine or fermented beverages being consumed dating back to nearly 6000 BC.

Much of the driving force behind the creation of wine and other fermented beverages was due to the unreliable quality of drinking water. As time evolved, the use of these beverages became more varied as the civilizations around the world developed. Along the way, alcohol production became more complex. Wine went from a drink for survival to more nuanced uses, sometimes having to do with ceremony, sometimes having religious connections, sometimes as a growing trade commodity and regional agricultural industry.

What all of these early cultures found out was that a stable, safe drinking source was vital to their survival. Techniques became more consistent and dependable as time evolved.

CHAPTER 2

Each region experimented with various growing and producing methods; all centered around regional resources. Grape varietals, climate, soil and storage issues were all important parts of the early production of wine. Not much has changed since that time. The net result that wine and other fermented beverages produce alcohol is no small reason for the continued development of styles and flavors in winemaking.

Throughout history, the pleasurable effect wine has had on people has much to do with it remaining with us as civilizations developed. People liked the way it tasted and how they felt drinking it. The notion of moderation and restraint that is justly advised within these pages, is a notion that could never have powered the enthusiastic development of wine as a drink of choice. It grew as a commodity because of the effect it had on people.

That being said, the tone of these pages will continue to emphasize restraint and moderation when it comes to wine consumption. Though there are certainly documented positive health benefits found in many of the chemical compounds in wine, they are outweighed by the adverse dangers of alcohol abuse.

The science behind the health benefits of wine is quite extensive. There are hundreds of articles available with lots of in-depth information about all the beneficial elements and compounds that are found in grapes. We don't want to make this book a scientific journal, reviewing the complexities of the scientific analysis. We have researched many of the outstanding writings on the subject and have come to the conclusion that the benefits of wine are much more suggestive than they are definitive. The science suggests a 'path' to follow not an order.

Drinking wine in and of itself will not make you a healthier person. There. We said it. There is no magic pill found in wine that will make THE difference in your personal quest for better health. We suspect you may have known that, but we don't want you to think we are offering up some form of snake oil here.

But, there are very specific elements found in fermented grape juice and, more specifically, grape skins that have clear health benefits. The majority of the scientific work keeps coming back to the presence of the compound resveratrol in grape skins, and the effect that *polyphenol* has on the circulatory system. There have been numerous studies showing that Resveratrol has a profound ability to fight certain forms of cancer. It also has been shown to have an ability to aid better blood HDL-cholesterol and vascular function. The anti-oxidants in the grape skins with high percentages of Resveratrol have also been shown to aid in reducing the chance of stroke and certain types of diabetes.

Resveratrol is a compound that is found in varying degrees in a variety of fruits, most especially red grapes. There are some grapes that have higher percentages of the compound, as well. Some of those grape varietals (Cabernet Franc) are easier to find in the marketplace. Cabernet Franc-based wines are traditionally found in red wines from France's Loire Valley but the grape is grown in many other places including Northern Italy and North America. Some of the grape varietals with high percentages of resveratrol are not so easy to find in the average wine shop. Rkatsiteli is a grape grown in the Finger Lakes of New York. It has some of the highest amounts of this compound found in any grapes. The wine made from that grape is much more difficult to find, but worth hunting down. It is quite tasty.

What most of the wines (red and white) with highest percentages of the compound have in common is that they are usually found in cooler growing areas. Most of the evidence shows that climate has an effect on the amount of the compound found in the grape skins. For example, Finger Lake (NY) Pinot Noirs have significantly higher amounts of resveratrol than those from warmer climate versions like California or some regions in France.

What are the reasons that cooler climate wines (reds, mostly) have this added edge? Think agriculture. Think taking things slowly and deliberately. The ripening of the grapes in cooler climates happens at a more relaxed, less full-throttle speed. The grapes have time to develop their potential over a longer arc. The skins have less of a chance of getting over-cooked, thus burning out some of the total characteristics of the whole fruit. This varies from grape varietal to grape varietal but the context is clear. Climate makes a difference in the structural makeup of agricultural products. That makes sense, right?

In a cooler climate, not all grape varietals can thrive. They may get planted at some wineries, but the results are usually not very pleasing to the average wine drinker. Cool climates might not allow full ripening of some grapes. If the grapes don't get ripe, there may be bitter, sour, vegetal (green) flavors some might not prefer. Sometimes the wineries in those areas will add some sweetening agents to counteract this higher acidic profile. And there is nothing 'wrong' with that. Their goal is to make something enjoyable with the materials they have. But, grapes with those higher percentages of resveratrol thrive in those cooler climates.

It is up to the consumer to decide if the flavors of those wines are to their liking. Wines from these areas can be a little tart and unripe. The acidity levels can be high and the texture in the wines may be not as smooth as the same type of wine made in a warmer environment. These are strong generalizations. Winemakers these days are able to contort and mask all kinds of flavors with modern techniques. But they can't drastically change the levels of iron, potassium and other healthy organic compounds in the grapes grown in their vineyards, short of adding those things to their soil.

Turning knowledge into action

What we are finding with the knowledge of this information about wine is that it can become a very sensible addition to a healthier, more responsible approach to personal lifestyle choices. If this book has one clear message it would be about making better choices. Without preaching orders to exercise, eat better and look both ways before you cross the street, we are saying that you are in control of your path to a healthier, more informed lifestyle. The wine information here is clearly only useful if it is combined with better choices in all areas of your life. As previously stated, there is no magic pill found in Malbec.

The combination of better food choices, consistent exercise and, overall, more informed decisions in the marketplace of life is something we should all to take to heart as the years go on. Wine can be a very enjoyable and delicious part of those choices. The social component of how wine is usually consumed plays right into our theme. Moderate drinking of wine is usually combined with a meal or done in a social setting, be it a restaurant, a book club, etc. We don't see binge wine drinking as a popular drinking activity. Wine usually doesn't connote the atmosphere of a "kegger" or a Tequila experience.

Wine can lead to a more measured, mellow and relaxing social experience. There are many wine-related activities that can be explored, such as tastings at wine shops, with friends, or wine dinners at restaurants. Later in the book, we will get into more detail about some of these opportunities.

Our goal is to continue to suggest that incorporating a healthy use of wine into your life can be part of an enriching, pleasurable lifestyle. It can be a great part of savoring your experiences.

Action Item "Take-away":
A NOTE FROM THE AUTHOR

There was a temptation for me to provide a specific number of glasses per day you should or could limit yourself to. However, the more I thought about it and the more observations I made, I realized there is no clear answer here.

A single glass of wine at the end of each day is excessive for many people and a mere warm-up for others. Three glasses on a Friday evening is binge drinking for some, but certainly not all.

As with most things, there is never a "one size fits all" answer here. Wisdom is your best guide.

A brief story may be in order.

Several years ago I had some blood work done. My cholesterol levels were wildly askew. Apparently, one of those ratios of good cholesterol to total cholesterol was so far off, the physician I was dealing with at the time postulated I should be dead. Rather dramatic I thought, but a medical opinion none the less.

In order to bring this issue under control, I was told – in no uncertain terms – "I should drink two glasses of wine every day for the rest of my life."

I will do my very best to be compliant.

In summary, drink wine…just not all of it.

If you have to ask yourself if you want one more…you don't need it.

I hope that helps.

CHAPTER 3

Your Obstacles

"There are plenty of difficult obstacles in your path.

Don't allow yourself to become one of them."

- Ralph Marston

Objectives:

1. To understand exactly what obstacles stand in your way

2. To create the right mindset for battling the 4 major obstacles to your lifestyle success

What exactly are the things that get in the way of good health and effective weight management? Briefly, the obstacles you may face can be put into one of the following categories:

– Poor nutrition

– A sedentary lifestyle

– Disease conditions – which in many cases can result from a combination of the first two, but of course, many disease conditions are out of our control.

– Stress and other unhealthy behaviors

Let's look at these and clarify exactly what we can do to control each area.

CHAPTER 3

Nutrition

It's no secret. The typical American diet is atrocious... if you choose it to be. This is not to say a healthy diet is impossible in this country. Anyone can eat the right foods with a minimum of effort. So why is our food and general diet viewed so poorly?

There are a few factors involved here. In one sense, we are a victim of our own success. We are a country of innovation and production. Over time, we became extremely good at producing vast quantities of relatively inexpensive food. With this high volume, however, came a slow and steady decline in quality.

Along came the processing of our food...

Keep in mind: Food processing is done for the convenience of the manufacturer, not the health of the consumer.

Chemicals have been added to our food for a multitude of reasons; among them are: To prolong shelf life, to enhance flavor and to replace vitamins lost during the processing itself. The end result is food not as it was intended to be, but food that is quick, inexpensive and of questionable quality.

In his excellent book *"In Defense of Food"*, author Michael Pollan accurately describes how our approach to food has changed through the definition of what he calls *nutritionism*. We have slowly moved away from thinking of food as food, and instead think of food as the nutrients which comprise it.

In moving away from the thought of whole foods, we move away from the way we were intended to eat. In addition, we open the door for scientific analysis and manipulation of our food, as well as its processing and marketing.

Again, this is entirely for the convenience of the food industry and threatens our health in a slow and insidious way; a way approved by the government, who acts in lock-step with the powerful food lobby.

Keep in mind: The food industry is a business like any other. They are driven by profits, must appease shareholders and must conduct operations in the most efficient way possible. None of these motives are driven by the health of the consumer.

The next factor is convenience. We crave speed. We see it across our society. We want fast answers, a blazing internet connection, the quickest route to the office, rapid growth and expansion, immediate recaps of the day's events, etc.

CHAPTER 3

When applied to our food, speed is not a good thing.

While our days may be fast, food should be slow. This is a basic tenet of *"The Red Wine Diet"*.

Food should go beyond simply refueling our bodies with nutrients. Food should be thought through, enjoyed, savored and appreciated for its own sake. When we lose this aspect of the eating process, we are short-changing our life experience as a whole.

As we get into the philosophy of the *"Red Wine Diet"*, we will understand the need for food as a source of health, relaxation and enjoyment. I hope this mindset will start to change how you think about what you eat, apart from the simple ingestion of calories, and towards thinking of food as the essential center of your health.

Eating needs to be a mindful activity, reclaiming the importance it has lost.

With this philosophy in mind, I describe the heart of *"The Red Wine Diet"* as one based loosely on the Mediterranean Diet, with some "adjustments" that we will describe in detail in the chapters ahead. The *"Red Wine Diet"* definitely mirrors the Mediterranean approach when it comes to the associated mindset and social aspects.

To say that one diet fits all is a lie. If there was one effective nutritional approach which always worked for everyone, we would all be doing it.

People vary tremendously. Some require more protein to build muscle mass, others fewer carbs because of their weight loss goals. There are massive ethnic and regional variations. Therefore, we MUST adapt even the most proven 'diets' to suit individual needs.

There is an expression in strength training, credited to Louie Simmons, a famous powerlifting coach who said, "Everything works, but nothing works forever." In short, you should have some type of system or mental guidelines when it comes to eating, but these guidelines will change over time.

For example, as a teenager, you can eat pretty poorly – nutritionally speaking – and still stay lean. You have many factors in your favor; a rapid metabolism, muscle mass growth and peak hormone production.

It stands to reason that when these three powerful factors fade, eating habits must change as well. Let's try to put this logically.

CHAPTER 3

Most people eat a relatively fixed amount of food each day. They tend to stay with the same foods due to habit and preferred taste. Therefore, caloric intake remains fairly steady over the years. Also, we often do not see large swings in *activity levels* for most people. That is, they exert roughly the same number of calories each day and display the same level of physical activity. If you run, walk or go to the gym regularly, barring injury, your patterns remain fairly steady.

However, looking at the three factors above, we understand that our metabolism slows starting in our 30's. After age 40, we can lose ½ pond of muscle mass per year. In addition, testosterone levels and growth hormone secretion begin to plummet around the same time.

It is as if nature is telling us, "Hey, you have completed your assigned tasks (such as procreation, etc.) you won't need these hormones anymore." It is actually kind of disappointing to think about…

So what happens when activity level and caloric intake remain relatively constant and metabolism, muscle mass and hormone levels decrease? The result is what I call the "Fat Gap".

Let's say you start a given decade at a certain weight. If you keep your weight steady for 10 years, you could brag about your successful weight management to family and friends, and be proud about keeping the added pounds off when others around you have failed.

However, there is a problem. You are now five pounds fatter! You have lost five pounds of muscle and gained 5 pounds of fat. Going forward, this trend will decrease your ability to metabolize sugar. You have entered a downward spiral under the illusion of a steady body weight.

You must adjust your food intake approach (or significantly increase your activity level) in order to fight this insidious trend. Everything works, but not everything works forever. You must change your system and your mindset to suit the physical changes in your body.

When we start to see these changes, we need the clarity of thought to realize we are making decisions today which will directly impact our quality of life in the coming decades.

A Note on "Cheat Meals"

If you have spent any time reading about 'diets', it is likely you have come across the concept of the cheat meal. By definition, a cheat meal is a planned meal where the rules of your diet are intentionally suspended for that one meal.

CHAPTER 3

Cheat meals are generally found as integral parts of diets involving challenging limits of some kind. If your new diet relies upon significant calorie restriction, a cheat meal is essentially a predetermined reward; usually placed on a weekend evening.

For one meal, you are allowed to eat foods otherwise forbidden. There is a good bit of science behind this concept. If you use calorie restriction as a way to lose weight, your body can begin to slow its own metabolism as a way to preserve calories. Your body thinks you are starving and responds by slowing down the rate at which you burn calories on a daily basis. Not good!

In order to prevent the slowing of your metabolism, a cheat meal is a way to tell the body that food is actually still plentiful and hence switching over to starvation mode is not necessary.

Another justification for the cheat meal is to provide a mental reprieve from the preceding week's deprivation. It keeps the dieter sane, if you will. The theory says that if you can see a light at the end of the tunnel in the form of a meal without rules, you are more likely to remain compliant during the challenges of the week.

While some of this makes sense, let's be clear…cheat meals have no place in *"The Red Wine Diet"*.

Why? The above rationale makes cheat meals sound viable, doesn't it?

With *"The Red Wine Diet"* you can indulge to a small degree far more regularly. Since there are no prolonged periods of calorie deprivation, there is therefore no need for a weekly splurge. Small desserts can be eaten on a few occasions. Wine is obviously an option as well.

The psychological strain so common with many diets does not exist with *"The Red Wine Diet"*.

Much of the description of *"The Red Wine Diet"* mirrors that of the Mediterranean Diet. It is difficult to deny the benefits of arguably one of the most healthful nutritional approaches known to man.

However, there are several key differences which will be detailed in the chapter explaining the actual foods included in *"The Red Wine Diet"*.

A Sedentary Lifestyle

If nutrition is the solution to good health, one can view a sedentary lifestyle as the catalyst for disaster. A catalyst is anything that speeds up a reaction. Avoiding exercise will not immediately kill you, but it will certainly speed up the process.

We all know people who avoid exercise like the plague. It is entirely possible to get away with this mindset while young. However, as we age, all those who so diligently avoided activity over the years pay dearly as they age and slip into disability.

Yes, disability.

Over time, these folks lose so much muscle mass they eventually cross a line. This line is not clearly defined or easily visible, but it is there. Very subtly, the loss of function creeps up and can push us over that line. Once we cross into disability, there is little chance of returning.

One day a person wakes up to realize they have a disability. The disability, in this case defined as a lack of function, prevents them from performing many of their necessary daily tasks such as: shopping, climbing stairs, carrying, loading, dragging, moving...all the functions we were designed to do.

Independence is gone.

This disability did not come from an injury or fall. It did not result from some outside force imposed upon them. It came from neglect.

It is foreign to our body for our systems not to be active. When our society moved away from a certain level of day to day *physicality* to a lifestyle of leisure, the cost was severe.

In our modern society, many people have an inverted view of physical activity.

They view formal exercise as stressful trauma; something that could leave them sore and achy. Therefore, it becomes something to be avoided, since it is associated with pain. Humans have two very simple emotions causing this to happen: Avoiding pain and seeking pleasure. For many, avoiding exercise equals avoiding pain. They do not see any pleasure is regular exercise.

In reality, the inverse is true. When we cease physical activity, our bodies react violently. Heart disease and diabetes find a foothold. By moving away from what we were designed to do, and towards a completely foreign sedentary lifestyle, we wreak havoc upon our physiology. This is the true trauma.

Dr. James Levine, director of the Mayo Clinic-Arizona State University Obesity Solutions Initiative is quoted as saying, "Sitting is this generation's smoking." He goes on to summarize his research on the sedentary lifestyle this way, "Sitting is more dangerous than smoking, kills more people than HIV and is more treacherous than parachuting. We are sitting ourselves to death."

Good enough for me.

In the American workplace, staying seated at your desk, entirely focused on your work is viewed as admirable. If your boss or supervisor comes by and you are nowhere to be found, this is a problem. This happens in spite of the mounds of research demonstrating increased productivity resulting from frequent breaks each hour to get up and move around.

While a detailed discussion of corporate wellness costs and workplace habits are beyond the scope of this book, many companies are now realizing the cost benefit of healthier employees and encouraging more movement and activity.

The trend towards a more sedentary lifestyle can be seen across different populations. Recently my 15 year old son was enjoying his summer vacation from school. He woke up late, came down stairs and proceeded to sit on the couch and watch TV while texting on his phone for hours on end. I made it clear such prolonged periods of inactivity were incredibly harmful and counter to his athletic goals. However, with the world now virtually at our finger tips, it is difficult to motivate many people to simply remain active.

Back to the argument for an active lifestyle…

I can hear you now. You are saying, "Here we go. He said this was not an exercise book and now he is going to tell me how I need to go to the gym 3-4 days per week and run like a crazy person."

Not exactly.

However, we do need to clarify the definition of activity versus exercise. For most of us, daily physical activity has a vastly different form than it did only a few generations ago. We no longer have to hunt for our own food, plant and harvest our own crops or walk very far each day.

CHAPTER 3

Most of the manual labor is done for us. To combat this decrease in our daily physical demands, many of us trek to the gym, run on the streets or we do some other form of activity in order to mimic the physical exertion which was normal years ago.

The reality is, physical activity is a required part of the human condition. We have seen that a sedentary lifestyle is an assault upon our design and will shorten our lives.

As promised, I will not dive into a prolonged chapter about how to build workouts, and what exercises are best for you. I will provide a simple definition of what it means to be active.

Active is defined as: "involving physical effort" or "characterized by energetic work". In short, if you are active and healthy, you are able to execute daily functional tasks and have additional strength and energy available to deal with a crisis or emergency situation.

In short, you do not have to be fitness obsessed, but you need to be fitness *aware.*

For the average person, it shouldn't take too much exertion to meet the above standard. However, if you have been leading a sedentary lifestyle, things change. In particular, as we age, being able to deal with emergency situations can become a significant challenge.

As I mentioned, on average, we lose roughly ½ pound of muscle mass per year just walking around. Only if we are regularly challenging our muscular system are we able to combat this loss of muscle mass. If we chose to ignore this fact of physiology, we risk sliding into disability, as described earlier.

What are some activities we can do to ensure that we remain active, and are able to enjoy the quality of life we all seek? Here is nature's list of active movements:

- Walking is a category unto itself. Walking is far and away the most natural activity leading to better weight management, a higher quality of life and proven longevity.

  Fact: People who walk regularly live longer, and people who walk *quickly* live longer still.

- Carrying, dragging, lifting and loading, pushing, pulling, chopping and throwing. Notice none of these actions involve a weight room. These actions are what we were designed to do. In addition to our brains, we were given a machine pretty well adapted to all these movements.

While we are here to focus on weight management, if you can find some way to include these activities into your life, your body will thank you. As someone who enjoys chopping wood on occasion and generally doing plenty of outside activities, I will admit, these types of activities provide me with considerable satisfaction. I have no real explanation beyond the fact that these movements are more natural, but yet involve movement in all different directions, making them more challenging and tiring. Yet they leave me feeling stronger and more invigorated.

Exercise, in my opinion, is a more structured program sometimes involving specialized physical activity and equipment designed to provide a specific result.

One example is lifting weights. With time, man moved from a rugged rural lifestyle to a more city-based lifestyle. Machines were developed to perform manual labor with more speed and power than man could possibly provide. As a result, we began to live a less physical existence. While some see this as progress, our bodies disagree.

With the industrial revolution, we ushered in the era of the sedentary human, and we continue to pay the price.

Without prescribing exercise itself, one powerful suggestion I'd make would be to bring back the nearly forgotten habit of a post-meal walk. This time can be used to reconnect with friends and family, enjoy the outdoors and aid in the digestion of a healthful meal.

Such an activity fits the "disruption" theme quite perfectly.

Stress

Visualize yourself in the time of pre-historic man. Predators were a real threat and life was a day-to-day struggle. While these early humans did not have deadlines to meet, financial worries, or live with the frantic pace we experience today, these were definitely periods of brief, life-threatening stress.

This may have been in the form of an attack by a predator. Escape from this predator or enemy group resulted in a period of what is called 'acute stress'. Our bodies helped up though these periods by pumping adrenaline into our bloodstreams raising our heart rates and even our strength levels.

CHAPTER 3

Once the threat passed, stress levels lowered and we returned to a relatively calm state. In modern time, being the creative beings that we are, we have figured out a way make stress an ongoing phenomenon. We have created 'chronic stress'.

We've created one of the deadliest conditions man has ever known.

Today, the feeling of stress goes hand-in-hand with a sense of our time and energy not being within our control. However, I want to dispute the "I don't have time" excuse right away! How can I get away with this?

Because we're all busy! Everyone is busy. In fact, the tasks we accept as part of our job or family responsibilities will expand to the time allowed for them. Whether you are a single parent balancing work with raising children, or a busy executive running a multinational billion-dollar business, either way the job gets done.

I submit for your consideration that very few people have the corner on the market of over-scheduling.

But, because we all need to eat and do so on a daily basis, the excuse of not having time has no place in the *"Red Wine Diet"*. We all eat and we can all do it in healthful manner. The good part is, it takes no extra time in order to do so; just a bit of planning.

The term "mindfulness" may be overused these days, but in this situation when it comes to stress and eating, it is invaluable. By simply being more aware of how we eat and by doing it in a more healthful manner, we become better at dealing with stress. Food, therefore, becomes a tool to battle stress. We can move away from stress-eating by using the "Red Wine Diet" as our tool to fight stress itself.

For many people, the pace of our lives has relegated our health to the back burner. People in my age group tend to have children in or about to enter college. They may also have aging parents to look after. As a result, people over 50 are often referred to as the 'sandwich' generation; being squeezed financially from all sides. This becomes an enormous source of stress. Additionally, they are likely in their peak earning years with long-term goals to be met, which does not allow them to take their foot off the gas pedal. Stress has become so ubiquitous, it is accepted as normal, despite mountains of evidence proving that it is anything but.

Let's take moment and look at some eye-opening statistics. I do this so we never lose sight of just how deadly stress can be, even when its constant presence in our lives can make us overlook the threat due to familiarity.

- 44% of Americans feel more stressed than they did 5 years ago

- 1 in 5 Americans experience "extreme stress": heart palpitations, shaking, depression, etc., which may come in the form of a panic attack, leaving one virtually non-functioning

- Work stress causes only 10% of strokes

- Stress increases the risk of heart disease by 40%

- Stress increases the risk of heart attack by 25%

- Stress increases the risk of stroke by 50%

- Stress costs this country $300 billion per year in medical bills and lost productivity ($100 billion more than obesity does)

- 44% of stressed people lose sleep every night

- 40% overeat and/or eat unhealthy foods

Source: The American Institute on Stress
www.stress.org

It is very easy to see how stress is directly tied into every other aspect of our lives from medical issues, to sleep deprivation, to diet and disease conditions.

Stress is as dangerous a killer as smoking, obesity, or even a sedentary lifestyle.

Reducing stress should be a primary goal for all of us. Of course, we all have stress on a daily basis to some degree. At times, we will also go through periods of extreme stress. These are unavoidable. But, successfully navigating stress is more within our control than we may realize. By not taxing our systems with excess body weight, poor sleep patterns and a lack of physical activity, we are in a better position to deal with excessive stress when is does come our way.

If you are active and fit, you can handle more stress. When you eat foods which improve health, rather than cause inflammation, you are better able to deal with stress. When you train your body and mind to sleep better (yes, you can learn how to do this), you regenerate your ability to handle day-to-day stress.

CHAPTER 3

One of the primary goals of *"The Red Wine Diet"* is to change these pervasive attitudes about stress, and learn how to utilize food and wine as valuable tools to reduce stress and to bring joy back into our lives!

I have been on a personal journey to remember how to have fun again.

I spent so many years accepting stress as a normal part of my day that, for a while, I literally forgot how to enjoy myself. Family events were squeezed in whenever I could, but the daily grind ruled my world. I communicated poorly, and often saw a person in the mirror whom I did not recognize and certainly did not want to be.

A change had to be made or it would be made for me in the form of illness or worse. Make no mistake – stress is one of the biggest enemies of our time, and may very well be the biggest obstacle we face in the quest for a happier, healthier and leaner life.

In summary, stress can easily make the claim of being the single most significant obstacle to your weight management challenge. Taking steps to minimize stress can pay enormous dividends. Stress itself starts a cascade of negative physical responses. Fighting these is now emerging as a powerful front in the quest for long-term health and weight management.

Action Item "Take-aways":

1. Pinpoint one area where you can reduce the amount of stress you experience each day, and take one concrete step towards improving this area,   i.e. morning meditation, prayer, deep breathing training, journaling, or spending 'gratitude' time.

2. Remove one item from your current nutrition pattern that you know is holding you back. Don't make massive wholesale changes, just pick one small thing and remove or reduce its use.

3. Add at least one post-meal walk to your routine this week. 15 minutes will suffice to start.

"Success is a sum of small efforts, repeated day in and day out"

- Robert Collier

CHAPTER 4

**The Basics of Wine I
– Jeff Slavin**

Objectives:

1. To define our starting point: The wine wines

2. To dispel the negative associations with one of their close associates…Rosé

A little information about the basics of wine can be of great help as you try to decide what you like and what you don't. Though we have touched on the history of wine and society, learning a little more about basic differences in types of wine can be a foundation from which to explore.

There are plenty of good places to learn the basic techniques of making wine. We will provide a source guide to some of those places if you feel the need to know more about fermentation, harvesting techniques, and the like. Our role in this book is to keep it simple and be a springboard to where YOU want to go with the information. We will offer just some of the basics to set a broad map to the larger field.

It all starts with the grapes.

Making the most out of the primary ingredient always makes the best final product. Most of the time, whether it be red or white, basic styles tend to follow a similar spectrum. There are all different shades and colors of wine that wind up dry, sweet or sparkling. The differences in those shades and colors can be found in the climate and the techniques used in the vineyards and in the winery. But the categories are usually the same. If white wine is something you prefer, there are styles and categories to investigate. They range from a light Pinot Grigio to a full bodied White Burgundy or a late harvest Riesling. The flavors range from a drier(less sweet) wine like Pinot Grigio or Sauvignon Blanc, to a full and more fruity (maybe more sweet) Chardonnay, Viognier and late harvest Riesling. How those flavors come to be is where the journey can begin.

Here are some lighter, drier whites.

The lighter types of DRY whites include Pinot Grigio, Sauvignon Blanc, Verdicchio, Muscadet and more. Each of these types of grapes can vary in style a little bit, depending on climate, soil and wineries techniques. However, the weight, or body, if you will, of the wine usually is consistently on the lighter side of the spectrum. These lighter whites are refreshing and versatile. Rarely are these types of grapes put into oak vats which might manipulate or change the texture of the grape juice. Keeping the focus on the crisp nature of most of these lighter whites allows those who like them to pair them with salads, shellfish, and generally, lighter fare. The wines hold up to mildly spiced dishes well.

Another great benefit for the consumer with lighter whites is that they are usually less expensive than most other categories of wine. The grapes don't need much manipulation. That is not to suggest that they are lesser wines or not as "complex" as other types. Nonsense. Many wines in this category are some of the most interesting wines made, in my opinion.

Inside of this category, and this will be the same for nearly all the other categories, the role of climate and winemaking-style plays a big role in the finished product. One of the easiest ways to feel more comfortable learning about wine is to throw off any notion of pretense that you might not be an "expert". You know better than anybody else what you like with regard to flavors. Wine is loaded with flavors and you may just need a method to organize your thoughts about it.

I always hesitate at wine tastings to suggest flavors or aromas to people standing in front of me. It seems that they want to hear clues that they then try to say "yeah, I taste that", when they really might not. Everybody tastes and smells and experiences flavors in different, personal ways. I feel it is more valuable to people to talk about the texture of wine which is more objective. Most people can agree on what is soft and what is harsh. Texture can be the 'mouthfeel' of the wine at the beginning, middle or end of the tasting. I also try to explain where the wine came from and how it may have been grown. Is it a cool climate red, etc.? That sets the stage for the taster to come to their own conclusions about the end result of them trying something new. It becomes their own discovery. I find that much more rewarding from an educational perspective than standing there as the so-called wine expert and telling the crowd they should be smelling thyme or rosemary in their red wine from The Rhone. Many won't. Many may say they do just to sound like they get it. Either way, the discovery should be their own.

If you think you are incapable of describing what you taste, I'd say you are selling yourself short. If you can describe what you like in food, you can understand what you need to understand about wine flavors. You can create a language all your own that is as valid as any paid wine expert.

Setting up a framework of your own can be remarkably simple. There are many ways to start the process. One great way to do that is to keep thinking about wine as an agricultural byproduct. Of all the factors involved in making wine, climate has the most profound effect on grapes. If you are in a cold climate you struggle and usually fail to make a wine that tastes like it is from a warm climate. The same goes for trying to grow Cabernet in Alaska. That grape needs a longer, warmer growing season to fully express itself. A colder climate Cabernet might be too bitter and vegetative for some. It can be done but the results won't produce a style that will be well received.

Therefore, when I'm trying to introduce beginning wine drinkers to a language framework that can become their own, I always like to talk about apples. Describing apples is very similar to breaking down the climate effects on grapes. My experience is that the public seems to have less of a shroud in their minds about apples than when they think about grapes and wine. There is some comfort level they have with apples that seems to disappear when the subject of wine and grapes is the topic. But the similarities in growing conditions apply to both fruits. Cooler climate apples like a Granny Smith are crisp, tart and have a light, spicy texture.

A warmer climate apple like a Fuji is rarely described like the Granny Smith. In fact, it tastes closer to a pear than a Granny Smith, in my opinion. The cooler climate apple doesn't get the same length of harvest, leaving the fruit a bit less ripe. That is a major reason why that apple is more citrusy and tart and the warmer climate style will be a bit fruitier and full bodied in style. Grapes are no different.

I'll pick on Sauvignon Blanc as an example. A cooler style of that wine found in New Zealand or France's Loire Valley (Sancerre is an excellent example) tends to be a little tart and crisp. They have flavors of lemons, lime, grapefruit and other zesty fruits. The climate in those colder areas doesn't allow the fruit to get ripe in the same way that grape might grow in a very hot climate. Cool climate Sauvignon Blancs have a freshness and vibrancy that make them great wines for seafood and shellfish presentations, dishes screaming for a beverage with bright acidity to match the briny, lemony flavors of the sea. Those wines would be smothered or muted by putting the wines in an oak treatment. Their high notes of flavor, if you will, would be lost.

Sauvignon Blanc grown in warmer climates is a very different wine. When that grape has a longer, warmer growing season the flavors begin to lean more towards melon flavors like cantaloupe or honeydew melons. The flesh of the grape gets a little thicker and the fruit gets a little bit riper in texture. Those wines are a little heavier than the cooler styles but not by much; but they taste very different.

California Sauvignon Blancs or White Bordeaux (mostly this grape) will usually not be confused with the cooler climate wines mentioned above. The warmer styles can have a silky, smooth texture and elegance all their own. They hold up to lighter dishes that might have a more intense sauce or spice. Where a cooler style of the wine would struggle with a dish that uses butter, warmer styles can keep pace. These wines can occasionally hold up to a little bit of oak treatment at the winery, adding to their smooth texture. Overall, there is no value judgment here. One type is not better than the other. You may like crisp and tart or you may like soft and smooth. Your tastes may change day to day or meal to meal. You know what you like best. You are the expert.

A few notes on other lighter wines

Outside of Sauvignon Blanc, about which you are now an expert, there are some other lighter whites to investigate. I'll try to use food types as the launching point for these wines. If you like shellfish and lighter dishes (salads, light poultry); Muscadet is the classic dry, crisp white from France's Loire Valley that usually gets served with shellfish. The soil of that region was a coral reef millions of years ago so the vines have to dig through a chalky mix that adds to the feathery, bright and briny style of that wine. Verdicchio from Italy's coast can also be a great choice but is usually a little more full-bodied than Muscadet. It is also a great choice if Pinot Grigio is becoming too light for you.

If you like spicy food like Cajun Shrimp or Sushi; Austria has a wine called Gruner Veltliner that works magic with these dishes. Fragrant and versatile. It has great body and crisp fruit flavors to match intensely spiced foods. Albarino from Spain, Vermentino from Italy, and Grenache Blanc grown throughout Europe all can be good choices of light to medium styles of wines that hold up to the heat. Some of these wines might be harder to find in shops or wine lists but are well worth exploring. As dishes get a little more heavy and the sauces or presentations use more fat (butter, oil, roux), the lighter wines may seem to become overwhelmed by the food. You can decide for yourself. If they do not hold up for you, a wine with more body and weight might be the next step.

More dry whites with more body

The great beast of the wine world for medium to full body is Chardonnay. It is very versatile and ranges in many styles. People love it and people hate it. Either way, this wine is very available and when done well, can be one of the world's greatest wines.

There are great, cool climate styles here that include Chablis from France's Burgundy region. Crisp, lean, a little smoky, Chablis is a wonderful wine if you are looking for a medium, but not too heavy white. Made from Chardonnay, some so-called experts think it is the most elegant of the rarely or lightly oaked versions of the wine. Chablis is amazing with shellfish but can hold up to heavier dishes with very vibrant core of spicy fruit flavors.

Un-oaked versions of Chardonnay have also become more popular choices of wine for people looking for a medium style of wine. They are made in all parts of the world and tend to be pretty good values. These wines are usually heavier than the lighter wines mentioned above and are great choices to bring to a party or meal where you don't know what to bring. They fill that great "undecided" category when you are shopping for a bottle. They may not be the perfect lobster wine or go the best with grilled chicken, but they will do just fine.

You may find that tasting those wines with those food types may set off bells in your head as to what type of sensation in wine you may find lacking or complimenting the food. You'll be making more educated choices the next time.

Other dry whites to try include Viognier (aromas of peaches and apricots), Chenin Blanc and Pinot Blanc, both wines with enough body to match bold presentations from the kitchen. Viognier has game changing aromas for some people. It also has the potential to be high in alcohol, so be careful! However, this wine has a bigness to it that holds up to bold flavors.

Dry Riesling from Alsace or white wines from France's Rhone Valley can also be great, interesting choices. They all have the "size" in texture to go toe to toe with "bigger" dishes. Casseroles or heavier poultry dishes like duck can be magic with some of those wines.

There are some slightly sweet wines that can be great choices, too. And there are lots of types to compliment plenty of your favorite foods. There seems to be a dividing line when it comes to Riesling in public opinion. Some people write it off as "too sweet" and think they should not even try or consider the wine, as if something sweet was poison, childish, not sophisticated enough or the like. Nonsense. Moderately priced, slightly sweet Riesling can be spectacular with spicy and fatty foods. The wines have naturally high acidity from being grown in a very cold climate. The grape itself also has a charming personality of flavors that done right can match up with heavier sauces and pork dishes like few others.

There is a sweet, salty characteristic to German Rieslings from the Mosel that screams for Asian food. Kung Pao, anyone? Secret confession....good German Riesling is my favorite type of wine, even the sweet ones.

Other good choices for slightly sweet wines include Vouvray which uses the Chenin Blanc grape. Though some styles vary, Vouvray is often found a little off-dry and rich enough to hold up to those creamier sauces that Pinot Grigio gets lost behind.

Gewurztraminer is another oddly named grape that can be a joy to discover and a challenge to pronounce right. Those wines have aromas that might remind some of dried apricots and honeysuckle. The wines are typically very spicy and can have a little charming sweetness to them.

Torrontes from Argentina and Malvasia from Italy can also be found in still and sparkling versions that have that little extra fruity sweetness to pair with salty, spicy foods.

CHAPTER 4

Almost any of the above styles can be found in sparkling wines. You can find lighter, dry styles of sparkling wine from CAVA from Spain, Franciacorta wines from Italy's Lombardy region and the classic bubbly of Champagne. These are perfect choices to have with appetizers and more. Some are as full-bodied as most of the still wines, especially as you start adding Rosé' sparklers into the mix. The sparkling category has a tremendous variety in styles and flavors. Price points, too. A general guide to finding your way into these wines is to experiment at the lower price points. Try some CAVA and then some PRosécco. You'll find they are quite different. How you navigate those differences will inform your choices the next time you go buying wine. You are your best guide.

I can easily admit that when I'm out to dinner and I'm not captured by any of the white or red wines on the list, I go sparkling. Besides the pleasing sensation of the bubbles, a good sparkling wine is a good wine, and that is what I was after in the first place.

And then there is Rosé…

Before the reader starts skipping to other sections in the book, scared of even being associated with Rosé, let the record show that these wines are as serious and delicious as any other style of wine. Don't be scared, drink pink.

Part of the fear, if you will, of drinking pink is that they have been viewed as sweet, syrupy, cheap wines, not worth serious attention. That may have been the case years ago and yes, some of those nasty wines are still being made. But Rosé can be a great wine in the hands of competent winemakers and there are magnificent versions all around the wine world. Like all other types of wine, there are many different styles. But first let's talk a little about the way it is made.

Red wine gets its color because it comes into contact with the skins of the red grapes somewhere in the process of making the wine. Without getting into specifics about the minute details of making Rosé, the key is contact with the skins in the process. They get a small amount of color because the winemaker made it happen. Sometimes they simply blend in some red wine, sometimes they bleed in some skin contact during one section of fermentation. There are a few ways to 'skin' that cat, but all roads lead to the pink drink.

If we concentrate on the pink wines that have been more carefully made, we will find some great wines very suited to different dishes and occasions. But if you like the syrupy sweet stuff, go ahead and drink it. If you like it, no worries. Again, you are the master of what you like. Tell your wine snob friends to take a hike. But being curious about the drier side of this life might be interesting. Yes?

Lighter types of Rosé are typically perfect with salads and lighter appetizers. They will have a soft fragrant aroma, with hints of red fruits.....the skins! They are the types of wines that diehard white wine drinkers should try if they want to venture into the depths of the big, bad red wine world. Come on in. The water is warm and inviting. These wines come from all over the world, using grape varietals like Grenache or Pinot Noir, but other grapes can come into play. There are French versions, Italian, Spanish. Price points are generally not too steep. They are usually fresh tasting and are best to be consumed within a year or two of the vintage. Some can age for more than that.

Good examples are from Provence and southern France but Rosés from Northern Italy or even Germany can fall into this category. Check the color. Most of these wines will have a light salmon color, a light inviting pink hue. Most will be as dry as any white or red from those areas but the fruit profile will be very different to the white wine drinker. A little more texture and spice. This mainly has to do with the tannins from the skins and the different fruit expression from the pressed juice. They may be too light for the heartier red wine drinker but they are a great compromise for diners having difficulty deciding between red or white.

The other styles of Rosé add a little more weight to their flavors and more texture to the mix. Rosés made with Syrah, Lagrein (Italy...find one), Tempranillo, Sangiovese may get to the flavor profile a regular red wine drinker might accept. They can be medium bodied on up to fairly full bodied styles (Bandol from France, Tuscan Rosé). They are great with medium spiced dishes, pork, sharp cheeses, pizza.

Though oak is not usually used in the process of making these heavier styles, you find examples. The winemaker may want to add the weight or spice that oak can impart. Some of these wines may be better with a year or two bottle aging and some can age for 5 years or more, usually the more expensive side of this category.

Back to the preaching podium: The notion that drinking Rosé wines makes you an outlier or not a truly serious wine drinker is garbage. These are some of the greatest values in the wine world in terms of not only flavor but the finding of the great passion of some winemakers.

A quick story. A great winemaker from Italy was selling a range of red and white wines to me. One of my customers asked if he made any Rosé because the range of his wines was so good. I contacted him that day and his response was, "I'll make you one". The next year it arrived and it was so well received that it has been sold out upon arrival every year he makes it. The point I'm trying to convey is that winemakers love making Rosé. It gives them the ability to have fun but be serious at the same time. They wouldn't make it if they didn't feel it didn't merit their attention. And it should merit your attention.

Action Items "Take-aways":

1. Never dismiss white wines if you are 'red wine-centric'. The summer calls for it.

2. Realize this is NOT the Rosé wine of your misspent youth. Try Rosé from this era…enjoy.

CHAPTER 5

Components of
"The Red Wine Diet"

"Wine is constant proof that God loves us and loves to see us happy"

-   Benjamin Franklin

THE RED WINE DIET

Objectives:

1. To explain where wine ACTUALLY fits in!

2. To understand the two most significant problems with the "Western" or "American" diet

3. To remove the "Addictive Foods" from your nutritional planning

4. To study the "Done-for-you" meal plans, grocery list and recipes!

When talking about how much wine anyone should be drinking, you drift into a touchy area. What may seem like a lot to one person is a warm-up for others. Culture, tolerance (natural or acquired) along with body weight and health status combined with past history all play into alcohol consumption.

I suspect many of us have seen that studies or at least heard about them. Some research indicates two glasses a day can battle heart disease; whereas other studies indicate that more than one glass per day can produce health issues.

It's time to put a face on *"The Red Wine Diet"* approach...

CHAPTER 5

Our first step, before we get to the actual food we eat is to list the foods we need to avoid and why. In addition, we can offer up viable alternatives to each so they are not really missed.

Being able to do this provides our first opportunity for a "disruption" of our existing patterns. We will plug in a healthier pattern where a damaging pattern existed before.

First: two simple concepts which can be considered the source of power within *"The Red Wine Diet"*.

P^2. Read: "P squared."

What does this mean? P^2 summarizes the lion's share of what is wrong with the American diet.

P = Portion Size

P = Processed Carbs

Control these two things and you control your destiny. When combined in a negative way, these two areas have an exponentially devastating effect on our health.

P = Portion sizes: As Americans, we have come to associate larger portions with 'a good deal' and getting your money's worth. It's as if being served huge portions at restaurants is the eating version of a sale at Costco or some big box store where we buy mass quantities of stuff at large discounts... telling ourselves we are all the better for it. Are we really doing ourselves any favors by cooking or ordering such huge serving sizes?

Of course not.

I recall an incident when my daughter was young. Our family went out to dinner at local restaurant which was very well-known and had been around for ages. This restaurant was also renowned for the enormous portion sizes they served.

On this particular evening, as we were being escorted to our seats, my daughter who was perhaps eight or nine at the time tugged on my sleeve and said – in a voice just loud enough to turn several nearby heads – "Dad, why is everyone in here so big?"

She was right. As I looked around, it was obvious that a disproportionate number of individuals were very much overweight as compared to the population you might normally see throughout your day. They were attracted to the large portions and it clearly showed.

This was the last time we eat there.

Were these folks really getting a great deal? If so, what was the real cost?

It takes roughly 20 minutes from the time we start eating a meal to when the signal reaches our brain that we are full. Obviously, we can consume quite a bit of food during this span of time. However, we can use this fact to our advantage simply by being aware of it.

If we eat smaller portions just a bit more slowly, we will experience the same sense of 'fullness' as we always have, while eating fewer calories. When done this way, we digest more easily, avoid the feeling of being deprived so common with calorie restricted diets and avoid the awful bloat associated with overconsumption. Make an effort to fill the vital 20 minute window with conversation to avoid excess intake. Simple.....non-stressful.....and effective.

P = Processed Carbs:

We are all familiar with the term 'processed carbs'. In fact, we have heard it so often it has started to lose its meaning and impact. However, the term is not always defined clearly. Let's use refined sugar – or common table sugar – as a prime example here.

Processed carbohydrates exist because, as a rule, they are easier for food manufacturers to work with, have a longer shelf life, and can be packaged in boxes, cans or bags. All of this makes such foods very convenient for the manufacturer. However, none of these traits contribute in any way to the health of the consumer. Avoiding these foods is a huge step in the right direction.

Bear in mind the old saying: If you grandmother would not recognize something as food, don't eat it.

We are not going launch into a prolonged discussion about how to read labels. While this is important given how food companies manipulate this figures at times, we are trying to encourage you NOT to eat packaged food altogether, hence the presence of labels should be at a minimum any.

The easiest way to think about this is to only select foods which have one or two words in the ingredient label. For example, is there any real reason for sugar to be an ingredient in peanut butter? Absolutely not. The natural ingredients are: peanuts and salt (and even the salt is optional!).

The "one word ingredient" rule will guide you a long way through the madness of the food label.

CHAPTER 5

A final note of labels. Food companies use a wide variety of alternative names for sugar. In fact, there are over 50 different names which can appear on labels. When used in combination, food companies can mask the true amount of sugar in any packaged product and sugar can easily become the most common ingredient in a 'food' even though the names used may appear towards the bottom of the ingredient list. Here are just a few of the major ones to watch out for.

Dextrose, maltodextrin, fructose, cane juice (dehydrated as well), corn syrup and corn syrup solids, maltose, sorbitol, and many, many others. An exhaustive list can easily be found on-line. Beware!

That being said, here is a list of the things you should avoid when following *"The Red Wine Diet"*. The "banned" foods fall into one of these categories: trans-fats, refined sugars or simply poor quality red meats.

At the bottom of this graph is a list of the unhealthiest condiments many of us use regularly. If these are a part of your diet. I strongly urge you phase them out! These condiments are a sneaky source of added sugar. Remember, there are always alternatives.

I did not wish to make this too oppressive, but virtually all of these condiments can easily be replaced with spices and other healthier alternative. I simply wanted to list the worst of the worst!

One final thought on condiments, obviously they are used to enhance flavor. However, you have to ask yourself, "Is this flavor change really necessary? Will this food lose all enjoyment without this condiment?" If the answer is no, pass on the condiments.

Addictive Food	Alternative Food
Cookies, cakes and candy (pretty much most commercially baked goods)	Dark Chocolate
Most pies and ice creams	Fresh fruit (without syrups)
White rice	Wild brown rice
White bread/rolls	Quinoa breads and sprouted grain breads (Awesome with extra virgin olive oil and a dipping recipe in the back of this book!)

Crackers/pasta	Limited whole grain wheat pasta
Potatoes	Yams/Sweet potato
All soy products	No alternative: Just stay clear of this stuff at all times
Beer	Wine! (White or red)
Soda	Diet soda with Stevia or sucralose
Condiments	
Ketchup	
Mayonnaise	
Tartar sauce	
BBQ sauce	
Ranch dressing	
Horseradish	

The above foods landed on the "Addictive Foods" list because they contain processed sugar or are wheat/grain based. The latter group is very high on the glycemic index and as a result cause a significant insulin spike. This sugar rollercoaster creates a pattern of cravings throughout the day which is VERY difficult to control without serious motivation – hence the 'addictive' label.

Sugar itself is a toxin. Never forget that. To make matters worse, it is an addictive toxin. The more sugar products you consume, the more you want. The same goes for wheat products. The more wheat-based foods you eat, the more you are drawn to them.

Mentally, you should these two foods should be closely associated as "bad options". Once you can engrain this association into your head, the sooner you can control the urge to eat them and the more rapid your fat loss becomes.

Here is a complete listing of the approved foods in the *"Red Wine Diet"*. Note the variety of foods available to you and pay careful attention to the portion sizes. You will see some of these foods in sample meal plans, on sample grocery list, and in recipe form as well.

Proteins	Serving size	Preparation methods
	Females/ Males	
Chicken	5/6oz	Plain, baked, grilled, or dry cooked
Turkey	5/6oz	Plain, roasted, baked, ground

Fish (non-oily)	5/6oz	Plain, baked, grilled, poached
Canned Tuna Fish	2oz	White albacore in water
Beef (lean cuts)	5/6oz	Roasted, grilled, ground
Eggs	one/two	Scramble, poached, omelet/skim milk
Cheese	1/2oz	Feta, Goat, Parm.
Smart Balance spread	½ tbsp.	Non-dairy
Peanut Butter	½ tbsp.	Teddy or Smart Balance
Yogurt	8/10oz	Greek, non-fat, sugar free
Milk –Skim/ Almond/ Cocoanut	1 cup	
Hummus	½ cup	

Carbohydrates	Serving size	Preparation methods
Oatmeal	1 cup	Boiled, Micro w/water per package
Kashi-GoLean cereal	1 cup	with skim milk
Couscous	1 cup	Per package instructions/no salt
Chick Peas	1 cup	"
Garbanzo Beans	1 cup	"
Lentil Beans	1 cup	"
Whole Wheat Pasta	1 cup	"
Brown Rice	½ cup	"
Whole Grain Breads	1 roll/ 1 slice	Pref. organic or quinoa
Whole Wheat Pita	1 6" round	plain or toasted

Snacks	Serving size	
Almonds	5 to 8	
Walnuts (whole)	1 cup	
Flax seeds	½ tbsp.	
Sunflower seeds	1 oz.	
Melba toast	2	
Raisins	50 to 80	
Dark Chocolate (plain squares)	1 square	

Fruit options:

Apples, oranges, bananas, Kiwi (1), American grapes (20), grapefruit (1/2), strawberries (1 cup), blueberries (1 cup), raspberries (1/2 cup)

Vegetable options:

Tomatoes...diced (1/2 cup), sun dried (1/2 cup), 1 whole

Avocado, asparagus, broccoli, cauliflower, green beans, mushrooms, onions, peppers, olives, spinach, sweet potatoes, eggplant, lettuce, kale, squash, turnip, cabbage

Spices and other:

Black pepper, red pepper, cinnamon, Italian spices, parsley, sage, rosemary, rubs for roasts, low calorie Italian dressing, oil and vinegar dressing.

Beverages

Water-lots, lemon water, tea and coffee (black or skim milk-no sugar), diet soda, Red or White wine.

You will notice several things about this list:

- Sweets are not banned in their entirety

- Alcohol is not banned (obviously!)

- Carbs (as a whole) are not banned

- Burgers are not banned

So what's the catch? Can you really eat all these things and still lose weight? Yes. You just can't eat all of them at once and in unlimited quantities!

We have mentioned that *"The Red Wine Diet"* is all about balance. Balance requires some measure of control. You can eat hamburgers, just not three of them and preferably without the bready processed carbohydrate bun, mayo, or catsup. Limit the number of burgers you eat monthly and track down a store that sells grass-fed beef.

You can have red wine, just not six to eight glasses at a sitting. You can have dessert, just not four slabs of cake. It's all about portions and balance.

When it comes to limiting red meat, some folks will have trouble. Many people eat red meat several times per week, instead of the several times per month, as recommended in *"The Red Wine Diet"*.

I remember when I was younger my mother would buy red meat quite often. Due to budget constraints, this meat was

– shall we say – of a lower quality/cut than I would prefer. Finally, the family made a request. Buy red meat less often, but when you do, buy a higher quality cut that we can truly savor! The food budget remained the same for the month, but the red meat enjoyment factor skyrocketed.

At the time, it may not have been as big a concern, but by cutting back on red meat by holding out for better quality, we were also making a better health decision without realizing it. A winning call all the way around.

Using an approach like this will increase your enjoyment of red meat; higher quality but less often.

A similar mindset applies to wine at our house now. We don't drink wine constantly, but when we do, I greatly prefer it to be of a higher quality. This way enjoyment goes up while budgets remain unaffected.

The Meal Plans!

Finally, we are going to present sample meal plans.

One of the reasons this approach is so easy to follow is that many of the foods you enjoy eating are here. You will come to understand that losing weight is much more about adjusting than depriving.

We are presenting two distinct sample 7-Day meal plans. The first meal plan contains slightly smaller portion sizes, and the second set of plans features slightly larger portions. You can think of Plan #1 as being suggested for females and Plan #2 for males, if you wish.

These plans follow specific calorie counts, but I have NEVER been a fan of counting calories, and I don't want you to be either. Counting calories and enjoying your meals seems to be mutually exclusive to me!

With *"The Red Wine Diet"*, you will not be tracking fats, carbs, protein or calories!

There are two major reasons for this:

1. You won't do it anyway, and 2) Doing so violates one of the driving forces behind *"The Red Wine Diet"*… enjoyment of food for food's sake. If you enjoy counting these things…and I guess there are folks who do…I'm certain this information is available on the internet. You will not see it here.

However, you **will** be tracking what *types* of food you are eating and *how much* of it you eat. That's it.

Keep in mind as you read these sample plans, in the next chapter we will be presenting a list of options which are designed to help speed the process of your weight goals.

NOTE: You will find your weekly shopping list after day 7 of this meal plan…used to apply to the sample menu plan. Finally, the actual recipes for these plans are all grouped together in Appendix A at the end of this book.

Wine Pairings

What kind of book would The Red Wine Diet be without laying out recommended wine for each dinner!

The list below provides two recommendations for each meal based upon Jeff's recommendations.

Meal Plan	Type of Wine	Country of Origin
Dinner – Day 1	Pinot Grigio	Italy
	Arinto/Vinho Verde	Portugal
Dinner – Day 2	Pinot Gris	Alsace or Washington State
	Gavi di Gavi	Italy
Dinner – Day 3	Any Dry Rosé	Various
	Pinot Noir	New Zealand
Dinner – Day 4	California Chardonnay	California, United States
	Verdicchio	Italy
Dinner – Day 5	Sauvignon Blanc	California, United States
	Gruner Veltliner	Austria

Dinner – Day 6	Virtually any Pinot Noir	Various
	White Roija	Spain
Dinner – Day 7	YOUR favorite "Pick of the Week"	Various

Side Note: My current 'house wine' – that is – our preferred pick of the week is Masi Campofiorin Rosso del Veronese

-Art

"Red Wine Diet" – Meal Plan #1: generally geared towards women (it simply contains smaller portions), but anyone can use it.

Day 1

Measure	Description
Breakfast	
1 cup	Instant oatmeal cereal. Fortified, plain, prepared with water and microwaved per package
½ cup	Whole walnuts, about 7 whole nuts total
1 cup	Skim Milk
1 cup	Strawberries-whole
Snack #1	
1 oz.	Soft goat cheese
1	Medium-sized apple (with peel)
Lunch	
1 cup	Chickpeas (Garbanzo beans) boiled without salt
1 cup	Cucumber, raw slices
1 tbsp	Lemon juice
1 cup	Lentil beans boiled without salt
½ cup	Mushrooms (raw, cut)
4	Large olives (ripe, canned)

1 cup	Sweet Bell pepper (chopped, any color)
1	Whole wheat dinner roll (medium, 2.5" diameter)
1 tbsp	Vinegar and oil salad dressing
1 tbsp	Smart Balance (non-dairy) spread
12 oz.	Spinach, raw
Snack #2	
1 cup	Blueberries-whole
5	Almonds
1 tbsp	Flax seeds
8 oz.	Plain yogurt, made with skim milk (13 g/protein))
Dinner	
1 cup	Couscous, cooked
1 tsp	Garlic powder
1 tbsp	Olive oil
3 oz.	Shrimp (boiled or steamed)
½ cup	Tomatoes, diced
½ cup	Zucchini, steamed
Snack #3	
1	Kiwifruit, medium-sized, green, raw & peeled

CHAPTER 5

Red Wine Diet – Meal Plan #1

Day 2

Measure	Description
	Breakfast
1 slice	Toasted, whole wheat bread (preferably organic quinoa…)
1 cup	Skim milk
½ tbsp	peanut butter (Teddy or Smart Balance)
½	½ large grapefruit (pink, red or white) fresh
	Snack #1
½ tbsp	Flax seeds
8 oz.	Plain yogurt, made with skim milk (13 g/ container)
1 cup	Strawberries, whole
	Lunch
1 pita	Whole wheat pita bread
1 cup	Feta cheese, crumbled
4	Olives (small-large canned and ripe
1 tbsp	Italian dressing, reduced calorie
1 lg. leaf	Spinach, raw

½ cup	Diced tomato
2 oz	Bumblebee white albacore tuna, canned in water

Snack #2

50	Seedless raisins
1 oz.	Sunflower seed kernels, dry-roasted without salt

Dinner

1 cup	White beans, boiled without salt
½ cup	Broccoli, boiled or steamed without salt
1 tbsp	Parmesan cheese, grated
½ tbsp	Garlic powder
1 tbsp	Olive Oil
1 cup	Whole-wheat spaghetti, cooked
½ cup	Diced tomatoes

Snack #3

20	Seedless American grapes

CHAPTER 5

Red Wine Diet – Meal Plan #1

Day 3

Measure	Description
	Breakfast
1	Banana (medium sized ~ 8")
1 cup	Kashi GoLEAN cereal
1 cup	Milk, skim
	Snack #1
1	Apple (medium sized)
1 tbsp	Peanut butter – Teddy or Smart Balance brand
	Lunch
1 cup	Sliced avocados (any brand)
1 pita	Whole wheat pita bread (large 6")
1 tbsp	Low-calorie Italian salad dressing
1 leaf	Spinach leaf, raw
½ cup	Diced tomato
1 patty	Veggie burger
	Snack #2
1	Kiwi fruit (without skin, raw)
8	Almonds

	Dinner
1 cup	Asparagus (steamed)
½ oz	Feta cheese
3 oz.	Salmon (wild, cooked with dry heat)
1/3 tbsp	Olive oil – pure
1/3 tbsp	Smart Balance (light, non-dairy) spread
1	Small sweet potato, cooked with skin, eat flesh only, no salt
	Snack #3
½ cup	Blueberries
½ tbsp	Flax seeds
8 oz.	Yogurt, plain, skim milk (13g of protein)

CHAPTER 5

Red Wine Diet – Meal Plan #1

Day 4

Measure	Description
	Breakfast
1 cup	Instant oatmeal cereal. Fortified, plain, prepared with boiling water added or microwaved
½ teaspoon	Cinnamon
½ cup	Chopped Walnuts, about 7 whole nuts total
1 cup	Skim Milk
½ cup	Blueberries, fresh
	Snack #1
1 oz.	Soft goat cheese
2 pieces	Melba toast crackers
	Lunch
1 cup	Broccoli chopped, steamed with no salt
½ tbsp	Olive oil – pure
1 cup	Whole wheat spaghetti
1 cup	Lentil beans boiled without salt
½ cup	Mushrooms (raw, cut)

1/3 cup	Sun-dried tomatoes
2 oz.	Tuna, (Bumble Bee white albacore in water)

Snack #2

½ cup	Raspberries
1 tbsp	Flax seeds
8 oz.	Plain yogurt, made with skim milk (13 g/protein)

Dinner

2 oz.	Chicken breast, white meat-grilled
1 tsp	Grated Parmesan cheese
1 tbsp	Olive oil - pure
½ cup	Long-grain brown rice
½ cup	Eggplant (cubes, boiled, no salt)
½ cup	Zucchini, steamed

Snack #3

20	Seedless grapes
5	Almonds, raw

CHAPTER 5

Red Wine Diet – Meal Plan #1

Day 5

Measure	Description
	Breakfast
1 slice	Whole wheat bread
½ tbsp	Peanut butter (Teddy or Smart Balance brand)
1 cup	Skim Milk
½	½ large grapefruit (pink, red or white, approx. 4")
	Snack #1
½ cup	Strawberries-fresh
½ tbsp	Flax seeds
8 oz.	Yogurt, plain, skim milk (13g of protein / 8oz.)
	Lunch
½ piece	Pita bread (approx. 6" diameter)
½ cup	Hummus
8 oz.	Minestrone soup-canned
	Snack #2
1	Orange, medium sized

	Dinner
½ cup	White beans, boiled without salt
2 oz	Chicken breast, white meat-grilled or poached
½ cup	Couscous, cooked
½ tbsp	Olive oil, pure
½ cup	Sweet bell peppers, chopped all colors
½ cup	Diced tomatoes
	Snack #3
1 oz.	Dry roasted sunflower seeds

CHAPTER 5

Red Wine Diet – Meal Plan #1

Day 6

Measure	Description
	Breakfast
1	Banana (medium sized ~ 8")
1 cup	Kashi GoLEAN cereal
1 cup	Skim Milk
	Snack #1
½ oz.	Peanut butter (Teddy or Smart Balance brand)
1	Medium-sized apple (with peel)
	Lunch
1/3 cup	Sliced avocados (any brand)
1 pita	Whole wheat pita bread (large 6")
.3 oz.	Garlic powder
½ cup	White Mushroom pieces
½ cup	Diced tomato
1 patty	Veggie burger
½ tbsp	Olive oil, pure
2 tbsp	Chopped onions

	Snack #2
50	Seedless Raisins
10	Almonds
	Dinner
½ cup	Broccoli, steamed
½ cup	Cauliflower (approx. 1" pieces) steamed
1 tbsp	Olive oil
3 oz.	Halibut, cooked with dry heat
½ cup	Long-grain brown rice, cooked
	Snack #3
½ cup	Raspberries
1 tbsp	Flax seeds
8 oz.	Plain yogurt, made with skim milk (13 g/protein)

Red Wine Diet – Meal Plan #1

Day 7

Measure	Description
Breakfast	
1 cup	Instant oatmeal cereal. Fortified, plain, prepared with boiling water/ microwaved per package
½ tsp	Cinnamon
½ cup	Walnuts, about 7 whole nuts total
1 cup	Skim Milk
½ cup	Strawberries, whole
Snack #1	
1	Kiwi, green, medium size, without skin
Lunch	
½ piece	Pita bread (approx. 6" diameter)
½ cup	Hummus
1 cup	Green salad with raw vegetables
2 tbsp	Italian low-calorie salad dressing

	Snack #2
1 cup	Blueberries, fresh
1 tbsp	Flax seeds
8 oz.	Plain yogurt, made with skim milk (13 g/protein)
	Dinner
1 tbsp	Parmesan cheese
½ tbsp	Olive oil, pure
3 oz.	Shrimp, boiled, grilled, or steamed
½ cup	Whole-wheat spaghetti, cooked
½ cup	Diced tomatoes
½ cup	Zucchini-steamed
	Snack #3
1 oz.	Soft goat cheese
2 pieces	Melba toast crackers

"Red Wine Diet" – Meal Plan #2:
(Men or larger portions)

Day 1

NOTE: You will find your weekly shopping list after day 7 of this meal plan.

Measure	Description
Breakfast	
1 cup	Instant oatmeal cereal. Fortified, plain, prepared with water / microwaved-per package
½ tsp	Cinnamon
1 cup	Walnuts, about 7 whole nuts total
1 cup	Skim Milk
1 cup	Strawberries, fresh
Snack #1	
1 oz.	Soft goat cheese
1	Medium-sized apple (with peel)
Lunch	
1/3 cup	Chickpeas (Garbanzo beans) boiled without salt
½ cup	Cucumber, raw slices
1/2 tbsp	Lemon juice

1/3 cup	Lentil beans boiled without salt
1 cup	Mushrooms (raw, cut)
4	Large olives (ripe, canned)
1 cup	Sweet Bell pepper (chopped, any color)
1	Whole wheat dinner roll (medium, 2.5" diameter)
1 tbsp	Vinegar and oil salad dressing
1 tbsp	Smart Balance (non-dairy) spread
10oz	Spinach, raw
	Snack #2
1 cup	Blueberries, raw
5	Almonds
½ tbsp	Flax seeds
8 oz.	Plain yogurt, made with skim milk (13 g/protein)
	Dinner
1 cup	Couscous, cooked
½ tbsp	Garlic powder
½ tbsp	Olive oil
4 oz.	Shrimp (boiled or steamed)
½ cup	Tomatoes, diced
½ cup	Zucchini, steamed
	Snack #3
1	Kiwifruit, medium-sized, green, raw & peeled

Red Wine Diet – Meal Plan #2

Day 2

Measure	Description
Breakfast	
1 slice	Toasted, whole wheat bread (preferably organic quinoa…)
1 cup	Skim milk
½ tbsp	peanut butter (Teddy or Smart Balance)
½	½ large grapefruit (pink, red or white)
Snack #1	
½ tbsp	Flax seeds
8 oz.	Plain yogurt, made with skim milk
½ cup	Strawberries, whole
Lunch	
1 pita	Whole wheat pita bread
½ cup	Feta cheese, crumbled
4	Olives (small-large canned or ripe)
2 tbsp	Italian dressing, reduced calorie
2 lg. leaf	Spinach, raw
½ cup	Diced tomato
3 oz	Bumblebee white albacore tuna, canned in water

	Snack #2
50	Seedless raisins
1 oz.	Sunflower seed kernels, dry-roasted without salt
	Dinner
½ cup	White beans, boiled without salt
½ cup	Broccoli, steamed without salt
1 tbsp	Parmesan cheese, grated
1/3 tbsp	Garlic powder
½ tbsp	Olive Oil
.8 cup	Whole-wheat spaghetti, cooked
½ cup	Diced tomatoes
	Snack #3
20	Seedless American grapes

CHAPTER 5

Red Wine Diet – Meal Plan #2

Day 3

Measure	Description
	Breakfast
1	Banana (medium sized ~ 8")
1.5 cup	Kashi GoLEAN cereal
1 cup	Milk, skim
	Snack #1
1	Apple (medium sized)
1 tbsp	Peanut butter – Teddy or Smart Balance brand
	Lunch
½ cup	Sliced avocados (any brand)
½ pita	Whole wheat pita bread (large 6")
1 tbsp	Low-calorie Italian salad dressing
2 lg. leaf	Spinach leaf, raw
½ cup	Diced tomato
1 patty	Veggie burger
	Snack #2
1 piece	Kiwi fruit (without skin, raw)
10	Almonds

	Dinner
1 cup	Asparagus (steamed)
1 oz	Feta cheese
3 oz.	Salmon (wild, cooked with dry heat)
½ tbsp	Olive oil – pure
1/3 tbsp	Smart Balance (light, non-dairy) spread
1	Sweet potato, cooked with skin, eat flesh only, no salt
	Snack #3
½ cup	Blueberries-fresh
½ tbsp	Flax seeds
8 oz.	Yogurt, plain, skim milk

Red Wine Diet – Meal Plan #2

Day 4

Measure	Description
	Breakfast
1 cup	Instant oatmeal cereal. Fortified, plain, prepared per package Boiling water added or microwaved
½ teaspoon	Cinnamon
½ cup	Walnuts, about 7 whole nuts total
1 cup	Skim Milk
1.5 cups	Blueberries, fresh
	Snack #1
1 oz.	Soft goat cheese
5 pieces	Melba toast crackers
	Lunch
½ tbsp	Broccoli chopped, steamed with no salt
1 cup	Olive oil – pure
1/3 cup	Whole wheat spaghetti
1 cup	Lentil beans boiled without salt
1 cup	Mushrooms (raw, cut)

| ½ cup | Sun-dried tomatoes |
| 2 oz. | Tuna, (Bumble Bee white albacore in water) |

Snack #2

1.5 cup	Raspberries
½ tlsp	Flax seeds
8 oz.	Plain yogurt, made with skim milk (13 g/Protein)

Dinner

2 oz.	Chicken breast, white meat
1 tsp	Grated Parmesan cheese
½ tbsp	Olive oil - pure
½ cup	Long-grain brown rice
1 cup	Eggplant (cubes, boiled, no salt)

Snack #3

| 30 | Seedless grapes |
| 15 | Almonds, raw |

CHAPTER 5

Red Wine Diet – Meal Plan #2

Day 5

Measure	Description
	Breakfast
1 slice	Whole wheat bread
1.5 tbsp	Peanut butter (Teddy or Smart Balance brand)
1 cup	Skim Milk
½	½ large grapefruit (pink, red or white, approx. 4")
	Snack #1
1.5 cups	Strawberries -whole
1 tbsp	Flax seeds
8 oz.	Yogurt, plain, skim milk (13g of protein)
	Lunch
1 piece	Pita bread (approx. 6" diameter)
½ cup	Hummus
12 oz.	Minestrone soup-canned
	Snack #2
1	Orange, medium sized

	Dinner
½ cup	White beans, boiled without salt
2 oz	Chicken breast, white meat
½ cup	Couscous, cooked
½ tbsp	Olive oil, pure
.8 cup	Sweet bell peppers, chopped all colors
1 cup	Diced tomatoes
	Snack #3
1 oz.	Dry roasted sunflower seeds

Red Wine Diet – Meal Plan #2

Day 6

Measure	Description
Breakfast	
1	Banana (medium sized ~ 8")
1.5 cup	Kashi GoLEAN cereal
1 cup	Skim Milk
Snack #1	
1.5 oz.	Peanut butter (Teddy or Smart Balance brand)
1	Medium-sized apple (with peel)
Lunch	
½ cup	Sliced avocados (any brand)
½ pita	Whole wheat pita bread (large 6")
½ oz.	Garlic powder
1 cup	White Mushroom pieces
½ cup	Diced tomato
1 patty	Veggie burger
½ tbsp	Olive oil, pure
2 tbsp	Chopped onions

	Snack #2
50	Seedless Raisins
10	Almonds
	Dinner
½ cup	Broccoli steamed, no salt
½ cup	Cauliflower (approx. 1" pieces)
1 tbsp	Olive oil
3 oz.	Halibut, cooked with dry heat
½ cup	Long-grain brown rice, cooked
	Snack #3
½ cup	Raspberries
1 tbsp	Flax seeds
8 oz.	Plain yogurt, made with skim milk (13 g/protein)

Red Wine Diet – Meal Plan #2

Day 7

Measure	Description
Breakfast	
1 cup	Instant oatmeal cereal. Fortified, plain, prepared per package Boiling water added or microwaved
½ tsp	Cinnamon
½ cup	Walnuts, about 7 whole nuts total
1 cup	Skim Milk
1 cup	Strawberries, fresh
Snack #1	
1	Kiwi, green, medium size, without skin
Lunch	
1 piece	Pita bread (approx. 6" diameter)
½ cup	Hummus
2 cups	Green salad with raw vegetables
2 tbsp	Italian low-calorie salad dressing

	Snack #2
1.5 cup	Blueberries, fresh
1 tbsp	Flax seeds
8 oz.	Plain yogurt, made with skim milk (13 g/protein)

	Dinner
1 tbsp	Parmesan cheese
½ tbsp	Olive oil, pure
3 oz.	Shrimp, boiled or steamed
1 cup	Whole-wheat spaghetti, cooked
½ cup	Diced tomatoes
½ cup	Zucchini-steamed

	Snack #3
1 oz.	Soft goat cheese
2 pieces	Melba toast crackers

CHAPTER 5

"Red Wine Diet" Shopping list based on the
7-day Sample meal plans:

Category	Food Choices
Beans, Lentils	White Beans Chickpeas (garbanzo beans, bengal beans) Lentils Hummus Veggie burgers
Beverages	Water, tea, coffee, diet soda, red or white wine
Breads and Baked Goods	Whole wheat dinner rolls Whole wheat pita bread Whole wheat bread Crackers, Melba toast
Cereals	Fortified, instant oats Kashi GoLEAN cereal

Dairy	Yogurt, plain, skim milk (13 grams protein/8 ounces.)
	Feta cheese
	Goat cheese
	Parmesan cheese
	Skim milk
Fats & Oils	Reduced calorie Italian dressing
	Olive oil
	Balsamic vinegar
	Lemon Juice
Fish and Shellfish	Halibut (Atlantic or Pacific)
	Salmon (wild caught)
Fruits	Grapefruit-bananas-American grapes
	Blueberries
	Raspberries
	Avocados
	Strawberries
	Kiwifruit
	Canned Olives
	Raisins
	Oranges
	Apples

Spreads	Teddy or Smart Balance brand peanut butter/Smart Balance Butter substitute
Nuts & Seeds	Almonds (raw) Walnuts Sunflower seeds Flax seeds
Proteins	Shrimp Chicken breast Canned tuna (white albacore)
Rice/grains	Long-grain, brown rice Spaghetti, whole wheat Couscous
Seasonings	Garlic powder Cinnamon
Soups	Minestrone canned

Vegetables	Cauliflower
	Mushrooms (white)
	Asparagus
	Broccoli
	Frozen broccoli
	Spinach
	Tomatoes
	Sun-dried tomatoes
	Eggplant
	Sweet potato
	Zucchini
	Peppers (any color)
	Cucumber
	Onion

Action Item "Take-aways"

- Prepare and print your meal plans based on the sample plans and recipes here.

- Prepare and print your shopping list

- Select a day to go shopping. To increase your likelihood of success, you should attempt to go shopping on the same day (or days) each week. This way even the food preparation becomes part of a regular good habit ritual.

– Experiment with at least one new recipe each week! This will add to your enjoyment of "The Red Wine Diet" approach.

What though youth gave love and Rosés,
age still leaves us friends and wine.

- Thomas Moore

CHAPTER 6

The Basics of Wine II
– Jeff Slavin

Objectives:

1. To develop a basic understand of red wine options

2. To make this whole topic quite a bit simpler

3. To look at the fun and simple **local** options available for further investigation!

The World of Reds...

If you're experimenting with the blush side of the wine world leaves you wanting a little more, you have come to land of the Red Wines and a vast world awaits you.

Red wine, as you have come to understand, comes from more extended time in contact with the red skins during the wine making process. Some wines see very little contact, but notably more than their Rosé counterparts. Some can see a much longer period of skin contact.

The effects are mostly predictable. The lighter side of the spectrum would include wines like Pinot Noir, Gamay, Grenache, all the way to Nebbiolo. But those wines can have greatly different types of texture and mouthfeel. There are many elements contributing to their differences, including the time in contact with the skins. The type of grape and makeup of its fruit can make traditionally lighter looking wines have very different drinking sensations.

A cool climate Pinot Noir that was gently pressed will taste nothing like a Nebbiolo from Northern Italy, though both will fairly light in color. Nebbiolo is really a very full-bodied red but for this section's purpose we are concentrating on the color of the wine. In other words, there can be a great deal of investigating that can go into finding the right lighter-looking style of red wine. The nature of the thickness of the skins can go a long way in sifting through the process.

Pinot Noir has relatively thin skins. That is one of the reasons that warm climate Pinot Noirs are a rarity. The thin skins and the nature of most clonal types of Pinot Noir tend to rot or roast in warmer temperatures. The truth is that Pinot Noir likes to rot in cooler temps, too. But warmer, more humid places have very little success with this thin skinned grape. A cooler, more sustained climate allows a more gradual development of that grape. Some other thin-skinned grapes will also have variations in success in different climates. Most do better in more moderate to cooler areas where the grapes can cool down at night and not roast in the open summer sun for long. All of these wines will have a lighter hue, ranging from just past pink for those lighter Pinot Noirs to a soft orange, red mix in Northern Italian Nebbiolo.

What most of these lighter looking wines will have is a more gentle sensation upon first sip. They may veer off to some exciting tannins (Nebbiolo), or a chewy, chalky flavor (Gamay), or a spicy, peppery, savory flavor(Grenache from The Rhone Valley). But they show the great rangeof lighter reds.

The Pinot Noirs and Gamays, as well as Austria's St. Laurent can have a gentle and soft side, with the Austrian grape leading more towards medium in body. The Italian Nebbiolo, America's Zinfandel (without oak and from cooler climates), and even Italy's Barbera can have a much more aggressive side but still not be as bold as a Merlot or Cabernet.

All of the above wines have a more "red wine" sensations than nearly every Rosé imagined. They will also be more properly suited to have with pork and meat dishes. Those complex proteins have some body and "chew" to them. My experience is that if the food has some chew too it, so should the wine. And these wines have some chew. Like other wines discussed in earlier sections, the lighter reds are also very much influenced by climate, soil and location.

CHAPTER 6

This combination influences the French term Terrior. Wine people use the word Terrior all the time as a summation of most of the natural, agricultural influences on the grapes and they are usually claiming that their wines express that Terrior. This might sound a little mystical and fuzzy. It might make a lot of sense. I'm in the camp where it makes a lot of sense. I'd advise to get less focused on the terms and let your taste buds lead you to wonder how it all comes together.

As you explore the slightly more gentle side of the red spectrum, you may want to take a few more steps to the end of the plank and examine medium bodied reds. The wines in the middle of the category are where most red wine drinkers find a sweet spot, if you will.

Most wine lists, most retail space on the red side is devoted to medium bodied reds. Here you find Malbec, Shiraz (Syrah), Merlot and the like. These are wines that are generous in their fruit and usually smooth in their texture. Lighter bodied-reds can be described the same way but grapes like Malbec have more weight, more noticeable, palate-filling flavors. The skins of the grapes are usually a little thicker, too. These are wines that can be made in a broad range of climates and conditions, as well.

The generous nature of these wines, with them not being overpowering in tannins, has made them a very popular category for wine drinkers. There are lots of different types to discover and the public has been discovering them at an insatiable rate.

In the last 30 years, the medium body wine world has shifted from Valpolicella and Chiantis to Merlot and onto Malbec. They have been in search of a smooth, silky and soft style that feels warmly satisfying. The comfort foods like burgers or pizza are especially suited to these wines. They are comforting wines, in many ways. They can be made in a fruit-forward, mildly oaky style seen in so many Malbecs from Argentina. They can be softly spicy Spanish Tempranillos that pair well with grilled foods. They can be sparkling, drier Lambruscos that match up with red sauce pasta dishes. They can be less expensive Bordeaux wines that use mostly Merlot in their composition. All are smooth and pretty soft on the tongue.

The wine industry has taken note and made significant efforts to keep the pipeline full and consistent. Techniques are very deliberately used to soften the wines including exposing more oxygen to the pre-bottling stage of the process and vineyard work that reduces harsh elements. The growth of plantings in vineyards of this category of grapes is always on the rise.

CHAPTER 6

Many less popular grapes get ripped out and replaced by the Malbecs of the world.

The marketplace usually doesn't spare the old vine, spicy and tannic Petit Verdot when the red blend of the moment is selling like crazy. Some versions of this Medium category include Chiantis and other Sangiovese varietal wines. Many are from Italy's Tuscany or Umbria area where the wines seem to be smoother every year.

Shiraz from Australia, called Syrah in nearly every other spot on the planet, can make lightly, peppery reds that sometimes get polished with some oak treatment. Many Zinfandels from California fill the bill as smooth, supple, richly fruited reds. Each part of the wine world will inject their own personality to the final product.

The European versions may be a little drier, but not always. The Australian and Californian versions may be less dry and a little fruitier. These differences may have more to do with the Terrior but many market-driven winemakers in this category seem to be trying to hit the very same notes. This is a very popular part of the wine buying market and some wineries look at their bottom line just like any other business. They tweak their final product to make it sell better.

This doesn't happen all over, but it accounts for a giant portion of the wine world. The red blend explosion the marketplace has seen in the last 5-10 years didn't occur in a vacuum. Cute labels with silly pictures of animals or the like aren't chosen because the winery feels they best represent their vineyard's unique ability to express itself.

There is no denying that the wines are joyful and generous. The wineries can be criticized as guilty of scratching that itch too much. But, then again, a famous musician once sang "Some people want to fill the world with silly love songs. And what's wrong with that?" If Paul was your favorite Beatle, go ahead and drink Paul. I think they are some of the best reds to bring to parties or share with friends. You are very likely never to offend someone offering up a red blend or value-priced Merlot. The wines might be a little loud with their fruit or spice, but not usually.

Is the category a little boring and predictable to me. Maybe. But that is just me. You decide and you will be right whatever you decide.

There are plenty of more adventurous places to find other choices in the category. It takes a little work but it may springboard you into the wilder, grittier side of the spectrum.

Helter Skelter. Some quick suggestions would be to track down some of those drier Lambruscos. Search out wines from France's South like Corbieres or Gigondas. See what the hell Pinotage is from South Africa.

Primitivo, Negroamaro, Mourvedre are all different parts of the medium red wine spectrum. Locating them may be harder but later in the book we will suggest some strategies for your search. These wines might be an area that you find yourself quite content. The range in wines is nearly endless and, when it comes right down to it, there is only so much time...

You may want more. You may want more spice. You may want more oak. You may want more tannin. You may want the wines to be drier, bolder, or heavier. What is a responsible wine drinker to do? Explore the Full Body Red Wine Section. That's what! For some people, this is where there is no turning back. Full bodied Reds occupy a place in the wine world where the meek do not inherit the earth.

Most of the other wine drinkers who favor lighter styles will balk at venturing too far into the Big Red Forest. Some in that forest never want to come out. It's all good. You will figure out what works for you. One of the best ways to figure out how to investigate this Big Red section is to find out where they come from and what good are they, anyway. Most of the boldest reds are from some of the oldest wine growing regions in the world. They have long traditions of growing grapes like Cabernet (Bordeaux) to Touriga National (Portugal). Most of the regions are in temperate climates where it gets warm in the summer and the growing season is longer than most other regions.

Full bodied reds need time to develop all the flavors they have, and a longer, warm growing region allows the full development of the grape. Trying to grow Cabernet in Northern Maine won't yield great results. The wines will be bitter and lack a variety of flavors, none that will be remotely pleasant. Climate and topography make a big difference with these wines. It does with all grape types, but this category is particularly sensitive to needing a warm climate to yield great results.

With typically thicker skins, these grapes are best served by lots of sunshine and then cooler nights, not allowing the grapes to continue to roast from the day's heat. Mountain vineyards start coming into play because they can be found in warm climates, but their elevation allows a natural cooling element not found on the valley floor.

CHAPTER 6

The color spectrum of these wines goes (most times) from dark to darker. Sometimes this difference can be found in the same grape type. That may have to do with oak's influence to the winemaker pressing more extraction out of the skins. Most of the time, it has nothing to do with price. There are plenty of very dark, cheap wines out there. Most of the time it is just the combination of the thickness of the skins of the grape, combined with the techniques used to make the wine.

One great exception of lighter colored reds but containing big, bold flavors would be Nebbiolo from Northern Italy. Barolo and Barbaresco, to name 2 versions of that grape are big wines that look more like Pinot Noir in the glass, light orange and red in the color spectrum. Some major areas where hearty red wines are made would be places like Bordeaux and Napa for bigger, bolder Reds like Cabernet Sauvignon. Cabernet is King for many liking BIG wines. It has a long tradition of making bold, structured wines that need time to breathe and hold up to the heartiest cuisine.

Cabernet holds up well to oak treatment, too. Most of the big reds seem to love the influence that oak barrels impart. Where Cabernet can have some peppery, dark and earthy flavors, oak can impart a pleasing minty or cinnamon toasty addition that makes some wine drinkers shout.

It may scare the hell out of those that can't stand the style.

The differences between Cabernet from Bordeaux and Napa has been discussed over the years, as if choosing one over the other is the biggest debate the wine world offers. I'll leave it up to you. Whatever you decide is correct. I can only suggest that both areas are trying to express a style that is well worth exploring.

Do I think that, in general, some Napa producers are trying to have their wines shout from the glass with the boldest of flavors? Sure. But, that's alright.

Do I feel that some Bordeaux producers want to have quieter, earthier wines that need more time to soften and develop? Sure. And that is alright, too.

As I've tasted more of each of the available Cabernets and Cabernet/Merlot blends from each of these areas over the last 20 years, they are coming closer to tasting more similar to each other instead of moving in a strikingly different direction. They may not be trying to make the same wine but techniques are much more similar and winemakers travel all over the world observing their competition. It is a great subject to investigate as a wine drinker. Be reminded though, that extensively comparing Bordeaux and Napa Cabs can be costly.

CHAPTER 6

There are many bold reds to explore and they aren't all named Cabernet. More available ones are Syrah and heavier Malbecs. Less available ones are Petite Sirah or Tannat and reds from Portugal's Douro Valley. Each will have a pronounced, chewy texture, with darker fruit, coffee, chocolate flavors coming into play. Some may be very earthy and dry like a Douro red using the grape Touriga National.

Tannat from Uruguay is an almost blisteringly tough, tannic red that needs plenty of exposure to oxygen to taste pleasant. Some may border on the almost sweet, black raspberry side of things like Petite Sirah.

Some California Zinfandels can be considered full-bodied, too. They have nearly sweet, darker fruit flavors and are usually complimented by the vanilla, minty effect of American oak aging. All of these wines are best served with hearty, protein-based food. You may not eat meat but these reds are perfect to break down animal proteins and match the chewy texture of fleshy food.

If you like venison or beef brisket, Big Red is calling to you. The chewier the food, the better a tannic red works.

A lighter red that has a light, soft texture will be overpowered by many beef or lamb dishes. The same applies the opposite direction where a cod fillet roasted in an oven will be overpowered by a Malbec from the Cahors region of France. But, as I have added from earlier parts of this book, drink what YOU want to drink. I can offer my opinions on food and wine pairing and that is all they are...opinions.

Once again, you are the expert.

And then there are the sweet, dessert wines.......

The best part of the meal for many people is the dessert. Some would argue for the dessert wines, too.

There are just as many types and styles of dessert wines as there are dry wines. To keep this section manageable, I'll try to keep it to the most available wines.

The history of the wines reaches back to the early times in making wine. The trial and error of making wine over time developed a sweeter side that has been perfected over time.

From Portugal's Port wine to Germany's Ice wines, the ability to make sweet styles is not limited by climate. In fact, each region adapts to their climate to come out with something truly unique.

CHAPTER 6

The warmth of the Douro Valley in Portugal yields super ripe grapes that are fortified (adding a little brandy to raise the alcohol) and made into a myriad of styles (white, ruby, vintage and more). The cold climate of the Mosel River in Germany yields grapes picked near raisin level at the very end of the harvest. Some areas in Italy will dry out grapes on mats and then press them into a sweet and tart style, depending on the region.

The bottom line is that there are tons of reasons to step up to the dessert wine buffet of offerings. Great winemaking goes into almost all of them. The great "Stickys" of Australia, Late harvest wines from Canada, Sauternes from Bordeaux; the list is filled with opportunities and adventure.

The best of the lot will have a balance of sweetness AND acidity. The sweetness is surely pleasing but if the wine doesn't have a touch of acidity and tartness, the ability to cut through the richness of the dessert will be compromised. A beautiful vintage port matches well with creamy cheeses because it has a great balance of fruit and acidity. Apple pie pairs well with late harvest Riesling because the wine can slice through the crust with a piercing tart component.

I suggest you try any and all of them. They can be reasonably priced if you remember that they should be served in small servings. In the $15-25 range, they present some of the best values in the wine world when you factor in cost involved to produce them. They are usually hand-picked at the end of the harvest, handled with tremendous care to protect them in this fragile period, and pressed and produced in ways that are quite different than the greater bulk-like process for many dry wines. They are worth every penny.

Wine Education Guide Section:

Earlier in the book we suggested that there are many opportunities to continue your wine education. Here are a few easy suggestions:

Find a good wine shop and start talking to the people working there. If you happen to find a shop that has an adequate selection of wine, chances are good that the store is doing regular tastings or has some kind of newsletter, online or in print. Sign up and show up to as many store sponsored events as possible. They are usually free and can be a non-intrusive way to get to know the people in the wine department.

A big question you might have is if your shop is a good one will be answered once you start asking them questions. They may know less than you and you may find in short order that you need more. They may also know quite a bit and become a great resource for your wine exploration.

The size of the store doesn't always matter. There are plenty of big box stores stocked with tons of wines but have very few qualified to answer questions you might have. There are plenty of small stores with what would appear to be a smaller selection, but find them to be rich with ideas and a perfectly acceptable array of wines. Your work is to shop around. Sign up for email updates, subscribe to some online offers from stores just outside your shopping area, too. Find out information any way you can. But finding that reliable retailer is invaluable. They are your true friend. If you can find the exact same wine for two dollars less a few towns over, your purchasing decision should consider the level of service you receive from your best resource, that great local retailer.

In support of the better independent wine store, a few words are needed about discount, big-box stores. Price is important. Price makes a big difference in many decisions we make in the marketplace. Service should be just as important. My experience is that many, if not most huge stores are inadequately staffed with qualified wine people. They pour their money into the price and the "look" of the store. They are owned by people who take your patronage for granted because they offer a sharp price. I would hope that the readers of this book, people trying to make better educated choices in their everyday life, would value the "whole" experience of buying wine.

Independent stores that care about holding on to you as their customer are increasingly aware of having good educators available during their busiest hours. Those retailers have to make your shopping experience a special one or else they are dead. They will get beaten on price and never know what hit them. If they can engage you with their selection and "value-added" services (wine specials, emails, classes, wine dinners), then you may come to see them as a true resource. I can't stress how important that free relationship is to helping you find out more about this adventure.

One can also find more formal wine education available to you. Local schools, be them college-level or continuing education classes offered at local high schools usually have some kind of wine education classes. Most times these are taught by highly skilled people with many years in the trade. The classes might not be free but at least you get to drink and learn at the same time.

CHAPTER 6

Sounds like a good deal, huh?

They will usually offer a range of classes that might explore a single region like Tuscany or focus on a type of cuisine with wine pairings. These classes aren't difficult to find online.

And speaking of online....the internet is a vast resource for you no matter what you are looking for. Magazines, bloggers (most have as much knowledge as you or less), online retailers, Twitter, Wikipedia....the options have no end.

I find myself using the internet to find out more about specific grapes or regions after tasting something new. Even after 20 years in the trade, new grapes and regions come to my attention. Online, I go.

I'd rather not endorse one sight over the other, since my needs are pretty specific and border more towards the technical side. Let it be said, the options are endless.

Endless is a good way to describe the scores of books and periodicals you can purchase. There are great, exhaustive encyclopedias of wine that can be consistent resources for the basics and beyond. There are monthly subscription-based periodicals by highly educated and influential critics and educators who might be more to your fancy. Just beware of what is projected as fact and opinion with all of these. There is no gray area as to where the regions are located or the where the grapes are grown.

There is plenty of debate as to what is good, bad and ugly. Just because Joe Wine says that a wine is worthy of praise doesn't mean you will agree. Be a discerning reader and critic yourself.

Action Items:

1. Pop into one local wine tasting. These event are usually posted on web sites for specific beverage stores or even on sites like "Meetup"

2. Try one red wine this month from a country you would not have normally considered

3. Have your own taste testing comparing red wines from colder versus warmer climates

CHAPTER 7

The Accelerators

"Small deeds done are better than great deeds planned"

- *Peter Marshall*

Objective:

1. To learn how you can speed up your weight loss through the use of one or more "Accelerators".

Before we get started in this chapter, I want to reiterate that this is not an exercise book. However, if you're looking to accelerate your results, there are definitely steps you can take to do that. Some involve exercise and some involve modifications to your nutrition.

First, let's talk about the nutritional changes you can make to accelerate your results. *"The Red Wine Diet"*, as we know, is a modification of the well-known Mediterranean diet. When you examine the Mediterranean diet-the true Mediterranean diet-there are two things which can be removed in order to speed up your results for weight loss.

Accelerators #1 and #2: Grains and Dairy – or the lack thereof.

The Mediterranean diet allows wheat and grains to be consumed with some regularity. However, by removing all grains from your diet, you will see faster results.

CHAPTER 7

I have had disagreements with many people about the value or lack thereof of bread in our diet. Consuming bread dates back to the rise of the agricultural period in human history. When a struggle for survival in life was a day to day physically demanding existence, it was vital that we had a very calorie dense food to supply the energy needed to simply exist.

However our lifestyle today is much more about leisure that it is about struggle. Therefore, we can make the statement: "Eating grains including whole grains is not necessary for good health!"

You may feel very strongly against removing bread from your diet. After all, we love bread because the taste is darn good! And when I suggest you give up bread as part of your weight loss plan, I am not implying that you must give it up forever. I am saying that you give it up only during the period in which you are trying to lose a certain amount of body fat. Once you reach your weight management goals, you can slowly reintroduce foods like whole grains on a somewhat regular basis.

Here's another strategy. This one is called "nutrient timing". If you must eat some type of processed carbohydrate such as good quality whole-grain bread, or even some dark chocolate or other approved sweet for dessert; you should do so immediately following some type of physical activity. The more rigorous this activity is, the better the results will be.

There's a timeframe after you do some type of workout in which your body processes nutrients differently. For example, if you consume protein along with some carbohydrates immediately after a workout or other exercise activity, those nutrients are absorbed by the muscles directly, to replace the energy you just used. Therefore, it is less likely than that these calories will be stored as fat.

Now we can see that when you eat your food is almost as important as what comprises your food.

The second food group that the Mediterranean diet approves of, and which we are going to address here, is the inclusion of dairy products.

Virtually all of my fitness colleagues agree that if you really want to lose weight quickly and effectively you will need remove two things…. grains and dairy.

The Mediterranean diet approves of consuming low-fat, high protein yogurt on a somewhat limited basis. For the purpose

CHAPTER 7

of losing weight, and in order to accelerate your results, you must remove all dairy....even Greek yogurt.

The goal of *"The Red Wine Diet"* is to provide a realistic, comfortable nutritional approach, which does not involve tremendous amounts of deprivation or sacrifice.

Therefore, you should approach these two restrictions *very carefully*. In no way should you restrict yourself to the point that you lapse in your discipline and go off *"The Red Wine Diet"*; and return to old, poor weight gaining eating habits.

So please keep in mind that these recommendations are optional, and should only be incorporated in order to *accelerate* your weight loss results, and not present you with a more difficult hurdle to clear in your weight loss journey.

Summary – Accelerator #1: Temporarily remove grains from your nutrition plan only until you reach a desired goal. In fact, add a serving of complete whole grains any time you reach a small goal along the way!

Summary – Accelerator #2: Temporarily remove all dairy from your nutrition plan, but only until you reach a desired goal. I would recommend adding a helping of Greek yogurt or even a small serving of your favorite ice cream whenever you achieve a milestone on your journey.

Alternative plan: Alternate removing grains and dairy on alternate weeks or months so you don't suffer deprivation of any kind, which could jeopardize your compliance with the entire program. This approach fits better with the overall psychology of *"The Red Wine Diet"*....this being a plan about a sustainable long-term approach rather than sacrifice.

Additionally, this could provide you with some valuable information by eliminating one food like bread and then a different food like dairy. You may be able to pin down which one causes you more trouble when it comes to weight gain. For example, if you notice that on the weeks you are eating grains your weight increases, or you feel more bloated, or have an otherwise adverse reaction to that food group, you've made a great discovery! You have found the food group that is your biggest obstacle to weight control success. That knowledge will give you the strength to slowly and surely remove that food entirely from your lifetime approach to nutritional health.

CHAPTER 7

Accelerator #3: Increase protein intake

This accelerator is incredibly important! First of all, it is important to see how this differentiates *"The Red Wine Diet"* from other approaches such at the Mediterranean Diet. Next, by increasing the amount of protein in your diet, you are replacing poor quality process foods with higher quality foods. One major benefit about increasing protein in the diet is that protein also happens to accelerate weight loss.

Without getting into too much biochemistry, a calorie is NOT a calorie...despite what one major weight management chain says. Yes, on a simplistic level, if you burn off more calories than you take in, you will lose weight. However, the rate at which you do so will be significantly impacted by exactly what types of calories those are.

Your body will treat 3 ounces of protein much differently than 3 ounces of sugary soda; kind of makes sense doesn't it? Therefore, by increasing the percentage of your daily food intake which is made up of protein, the faster you will reach your goals.

Again, this protein should be of the highest quality available. Lean protein sources include: Chicken, turkey, fish, bison, eggs, ostrich (seriously delicious stuff!), and grass-fed beef.

On a very positive note, the more we as consumers become increasingly mindful of the quality of the food we eat, the more common organic, hormone-free, and naturally-raised our food choices become.

Summary – Accelerator #3: Whenever possible, increase the overall percentage of protein you eat. Stick with only lean cuts of meat. Always eat the protein first when dining. This increases the likelihood that you will feel fuller without having eaten processed carbohydrates, starches or desserts.

Accelerator #4: Minimize fruits

This one ALWAYS gets people. Fruits are natural. Therefore, they must be good. Correct?

Not necessarily. If you are in a "transition state" where you are trying to lose weight, fruits are NOT your friend. Does this mean you can never eat fruit again? No. But you need to minimize fruit intake during your weight loss period.

While they are generally considered healthy, fruits are naturally very high in sugar. Some fruits like grapes, bananas, cherries, figs, dates and raisins are very high in sugar and should be avoided any time weight management is a concern. Most tropic fruits are very high in sugar as well. This includes pineapples, mangos and passionfruit.

Once you have attained you weight loss goals, it is possible to re-introduce fruits into your nutritional planning on a limited basis. As you have seen, there are fruits in our existing meal plans on a limited basis. By removing even these fruits, you create an Accelerator.

The news is not all bad with regard to fruits however. Eating fruits as desserts is a great way to cut down on processed sugar intake from traditional desserts such as cookies and cakes.

NOTE: If you are really craving fruit, try your best to eat them after physical activity of some kind to minimize weight gain.

Summary – Accelerator #4: If you have more than 20 pounds to lose, you should eliminate fruit – for the short term. If you have 15 pounds or less to lose, you should limit your fruit intake to fruits in the berry family such as strawberries and blueberries.

Accelerator #5: Walking and other forms of simple movement.

If you lead a sedentary lifestyle, you know by now that needs change. We have talked about walking before, but now let's get into some detail.

Walking is by far the easiest place to start.

As I've mentioned before, people who walk regularly live longer than those who don't. This is a very simple fact. In addition, people who make a point of walking very rapidly augment this effect.

Here is the best way to implement this accelerator.

When you go for a walk make sure you are alternating your pace with slower periods and faster periods. That is, make sure you alternate periods of walking very quickly, where you can feel your heart rate increasing, with periods of slow walking where you can easily catch your breath and you know your heart rate has return to a normal level. Once you've recovered, and your heart rate is back to a normal level, increase that pace again until you feel your heart rate rising.

CHAPTER 7

Monitoring your heart rate is quite easy these day. I strongly recommend acquiring a wearable heart rate monitor. Polar and Gramin make excellent products, and of course, there are many wrist watch-based options on the market.

This type of heart rate variation is far more beneficial than a steady-state walk where the heart rate does not go up or down very much.

One easy way to do this, if you're walking along any residential street, is to pick specific landmarks. Once you hit a particular landmark you can speed up your walking pace until you reach the next selected landmark. This could be a city block or certain number of telephone poles, a specific building, a street sign, etc. And of course, once you reach the next landmark you slow your pace down again.

This is also known as interval training. This is the type of training where you have periods of work alternating with periods of recovery or rest. For the most part, this is how humans are meant to exercise. Evolutionarily speaking, we were designed to run away and not become dinner, and then conversely, we are designed to chase something down and capture it for dinner and then rest.

Research has shown that we respond quite well to this type of structure. Interval training increases our metabolism and our cardiovascular fitness, and at a much faster rate than steady-state jogging does.

This is why I discourage my clients from doing any type of steady-state running. It is not the most effective use of your valuable time.

Additionally, I always recommend that people wear one of those handy heart rate monitors. In fact, I use one when I do my interval training. Based on listening to my own body, I know an upper and lower heart rate that I like to attain. When my heart rate increases to a certain level, I know that I'm being challenged. When my heart rate drops back down to a certain level, I know it is time to pick up the pace again.

Summary – Accelerator #5: if you are not a regular walker, please introduce this movement into your lifestyle. It fits perfectly with *"The Red Wine Diet"* psychology; offering time for stress reduction or pleasant conversation. Additionally, you are disrupting the deadly habit of sedentary lifestyle. Just make sure your exercise follows an interval type structure as described above, and not simply a long, slow steady-state walk.

This will significantly impact your results! Careful, this may lead to a desire to exercise even more!

Accelerator #6: Strength training

The idea of lifting weights is foreign to many people. After all, gyms can be confusing and judgmental institutions. However, lifting weights is as natural to humans as eating and sleeping. It is what we were designed to do.

A wealth of new information is beginning to emerge showing the powerful benefits of strength training, including outstanding protective benefits to our brains. Essentially weight lifting is an antiaging activity we should all be doing.

Few activities will provide a better return for your time by demonstrating what you are truly capable of doing, and how good you are capable of feeling, than weightlifting.

In keeping with my promise, I will not spend time presenting you with a list of weightlifting programs to attempt. If you are really interested in learning just how to start lifting weights, when you have never done so in your life, I point you to my previous book *"Boomer Blueprint"* which deals with this topic extensively, including actual workouts with videos and fitness testing.

I will only say that strength training, for many of us, is the key to weight loss, weight management and to an incredibly invigorating quality-of-life.

Summary – Accelerator #6: Start some basic strength training to build muscle mass. It is what we were physically designed to do. Again, for a completely detailed training program designed for adults, please see *"Boomer Blueprint – A Step by Step Guide to Longevity, Anti-Aging and Fitness for Baby Boomers"* available at www.boomerblueprint.com.

Action Item "Take-aways":

- Decide if you truly NEED an "Accelerator" in the first place. You can decide this by asking yourself these quick questions:

    O Am I already close to my goal weight? If so, it is likely you do NOT need an Accelerator

    O Do you have a VERY specific event you need to be ready for; such as a reunion, marriage, divorce, cruise, etc.? If you do NOT have a time constraint, I recommend avoiding the Accelerators. They may present more challenge than you need.

CHAPTER 7

- If you realize you need and Accelerator, pick the one you feel most comfortable with; the one you KNOW you can handle successfully and start applying it immediately.

- Once you have 'mastered' one Accelerator – this means complete success for 21 days or more – then you can try another Accelerator to keep the progress rolling!

In any moment of decision, the best thing you can do is the right thing, the next best thing is the wrong thing, and the worst thing you can do is nothing.

- Theodore Roosevelt

EPILOGUE

This collection of "actions" listed below – not laws or simple recommendations – are backed by science. They are not my opinion, nor are they simply guesses. If you are looking for a place to start, here it is. Come back to this list when you stray too far from the path to long-term health. These habits also happen to fit perfectly with the mindset and 'demands' of "The Red Wine Diet".

These 9 Actions first appeared in my book "Boomer Blueprint" (please see www.boomerblueprint.com for full details) and have only become more accurate with time, science and your success…

9 Actions to Help You Live Longer

1. **Run and walk quickly.** Studies have shown that people who walk faster live longer. It's just that simple. When out walking, be mindful of your pace. If you find yourself slowing down, make a conscious effort to increase your speed. Also, structure your walks and runs to alternate speed. It is important to avoid "steady-state" activity. Speed up and then slow down. Once your heart rate lowers, speed up again. Always alternate your pace for better heart health.

2. **Learn constantly.** Always challenge the brain. The day you stop learning is the day you start to lose brain function. Cognitive skill is like any other physical trait; if you don't use it, you will lose it. Brain stimulating examples include: learning chess, doing the crossword puzzle daily, reading or writing fiction or non-fiction outside of your usual genre, attending a book reading or presentation/seminar, taking in a stage play or concert, traveling to a unique destination with a different culture, etc.

   ABT = Always Be Thinking!

3. **Sleep restfully.** Human beings were designed for seven to eight hours of sleep in a 24 hour period. People who get six or less hours of sleep per night, generally have a higher body weight than their counterparts. The trend in our society provides a myriad of distractions to keep us awake. Calming the brain at the end of the day is the first step to better sleep and is one many of us overlook. If you wake frequently, find the source of the disruption and research ways to overcome this. If you do not sleep restfully, you simply will not be firing on all cylinders. NOTE: There is new evidence of a nightly process whereby the brain 'cleans out' waste products and toxins. Interruption to sleep disrupts this process.

4. **Interact with others daily.** Be social and remain social. People with a vibrant social network are also shown to live longer than those who exist in relative isolation.

5. **Eat colorfully and sparingly.** This requires some explanation. Your goal should be to eat a wide range from the color palette; reds, greens, etc. Work towards an entire assortment of colors. This includes a wide range of fruits and vegetables. I have heard it phrased this way: "Avoid the white foods: bread, rice, cereal, pasta, crackers, etc." Refined foods tend to lack vibrant color, unless this color is artificially introduced. Think: Mediterranean-style Diet.

   The second part of the equation is to eat sparingly. Studies have shown that – up to a point - the less caloric intake you have, the longer you will live. In short, be aware of your portion sizes. Using smaller dinner plates actually does work.

   NOTE: This does NOT apply to individuals whose caloric intake is already drastically low due to illness or frailty. Always follow your medical profession advice and recommendations.

6. **Lift weights religiously.** Nothing has been shown to retain or even gain muscle mass better than resistance training, that's just a fact. Running and walking only won't do it and yoga won't do it. These activities have their place in a healthy lifestyle, but not as the sole source of exercise. It is important to realize that every year, after the age of forty, you can lose up to a half pound of muscle mass per year. The only way to combat this atrophy is with resistance training.

7. **Worship and/or meditate regularly.** The inner peace that comes with these actions acts as a form of stress reduction. This is vital for a longer life and proper functioning. Whether you find contentment through church, Tai Chi, temple, or some other form of worship or meditation; attention to the needs of the 'soul', if you will, is vital for longevity.

8. **Stand up and lie down smoothly.** Move! Do so efficiently and often. In our modern lives, it is not uncommon to go entire days or even weeks with mobility limited to laying down, sitting in a chair, and standing up a few times, walking a little bit, perhaps navigating the occasional short flight of stairs and then laying down again. Studies have shown that people who

have the mobility, agility, and relative body strength to go from a standing position down to a seated position on the floor, then get all the way back up smoothly with minimal support or excessive effort live longer than those who struggle with this simple task. Stay mobile.

Best Quote: *"Sitting is this generation's smoking."*

9. **Reduce all forms of inflammation, diligently.** More and more research is coming out saying that inflammation is at the center of many diseases; with links to Alzheimer's, heart disease, diabetes, and more. The common link connects back to inflammation. This does not mean that you should take anti-inflammatory drugs constantly. Investigate the list of foods which have an anti-inflammatory action in the body. Reducing inflammation can be accomplished through diet and exercise.

APPENDIX

A

RECIPES

Delicious Oatmeal Atole

Ingredients:

1/2 Cup oat flakes, raw

2/3 Cup of water

1/2 Cup of milk – skim no fat

10 Nuts, walnuts, english

1 Cup of fresh strawberries

Cinnamon

Directions:

Place water and raw oats In a saucepan. Boil for seven minutes, stirring occasionally. Add the milk and one Splenda envelope. Boil for another two minutes, keep stirring. Remove from heat and cover until serving.

Serve hot or cold with cinnamon, chopped walnuts and garnish with fresh strawberries.

APPENDIX A

Summer Salad

Ingredients:

1/4 Cup chickpeas, cooked

1/4 Cup lentils, cooked

1 Cup mushrooms, sliced

1/2 Cup red bell pepper, chopped

1/2 Cup raw cucumber, chopped

1 Cup fresh spinach, raw

4 Kalamata olives

1 Tbsp. parsley, chopped

Salt

Pepper

1 Tbsp. homemade Italian salad dressing (*)

Directions:

(*) Homemade Italian salad dressing: 120ml. extra-virgin olive oil, 40 ml. red wine vinegar 1 tbsp. dried oregano. Place all in a jar. Shake well before use.

Directions: Chickpeas: Wash in water. Soak for 24 hours (change the water after 12 hours). Wash again and cook in a covered saucepan for 3 or 4 hours without salt, or 45 minutes in a pressure cooker.

Lentils: Wash in water. Soak for a few hours (2 are enough). Cook for one and a half hours without salt.

Both grains can be frozen for use in other meals.

Place the first six ingredients in a bowl, add salt and pepper, and mix gently. Place the parsley and olives on the top, and sprinkle with the salad dressing.

Couscous and Shrimp Salad

Ingredients:

½ Cup cooked couscous

½ cup peeled shrimp

½ Cup tomato, diced

½ Cup Zucchini, boiled and dried, diced (*)

1 tbsp. parsley, chopped

½ tbsp. extra-virgin olive oil

½ tbsp. garlic powder

Salt

Pepper

(*) Zucchini (cook for 5 min.)

Directions:

Cook the couscous per package directions.

Mix shrimp in a bowl with some salt, pepper and garlic powder. Heat Olive Oil spray in a wok, add shrimp. Heat for no more than 20 seconds. Set aside on plate.

In the wok place the zucchini, tomato and finally couscous. (Add a little more olive oil spray if necessary). Stir for 3 or 4 minutes. Add shrimp and remove from heat. Plate mixture and sprinkle some parsley on the top and serve.

Tip:

The best Extra-virgin Olive Oil comes in a dark glass bottle and must be kept in a dark place.

Chicken and Avocado Wraps

Ingredients:

1/2 Cup chicken breast, cooked, chopped

1/2 Cup raw avocado, diced

1 tbsp. coriander, chopped

1/2 Tbsp. red onion, chopped

1/2 Tsp. extra-virgin olive oil

Salt

1 Whole-wheat wrap

Directions:

Place the avocado in a bowl with coriander, onion, a little salt and olive oil. Mix gently. You can add some red wine vinegar drops.

Heat a grill pan and add wrap. Warm it in both sides.

Place the wrap on plate and add salad and cooked chicken. Wrap it.

Greek Tuna Salad

Ingredients:

3 Oz. can tuna in water	1Piece whole-wheat pita bread
½ Cup feta cheese	1Tbsp. homemade Italian salad dressing
6 Black Greek olives	1 Pinch of thyme
1/4 Cup tomato, diced	Salt
½ Cup fresh spinach, chopped	Pepper

Directions:

Place drained tuna in a glass bowl, crumble with a fork.

Place spinach (Spinach should be cut with a plastic knife).

Add the tomatoes, olives, thyme and cheese. Mix carefully and add some salt, pepper and the homemade Italian salad dressing.

Fettuccine and Broccoli

Ingredients:

1 Cup whole-wheat fettuccine, cooked	½ Tbsp. extra-virgin olive oil
½ Cup broccoli, cooked & drained	Pepper
1 Tbsp. parmesan cheese, grated	Oregano
1/2 Tbsp. garlic powder	Salt
½ Cup tomato, diced	

Directions:

Heat olive oil spray in a medium pan over medium heat. Add broccoli, tomatoes and sprinkle some garlic powder, pepper and salt. Heat for about 3 minutes.

Add Fettuccine and heat up. Remove from heat, and transfer to the plate.

Sprinkle with Olive Oil, oregano, and finally the grated parmesan cheese.

You can add 1/2 cup of boiled white beans to this recipe along with tomatoes and broccoli.

Mediterranean Omelet

Ingredients:

1 Slice whole-wheat bread, toasted	1 tbsp. extra-virgin olive oil
2 Eggs	Salt
1 Small tomato, sliced	Pepper
2 White mushrooms, sliced	Oregano

Directions:

Cut tomatoes and mushrooms in thin slices. Heat olive oil spray in a medium non-stick pan over medium heat. Add the tomatoes and mushrooms. Cook for about two minutes stirring. Season with salt, pepper, and oregano & set aside. Meanwhile, in a small bowl beat together the eggs, add one tablespoon of cold water and season with salt and pepper.

Heat the olive oil in a 20" non-stick pan over medium heat & add eggs. Cook with low to medium heat until the bottom is golden. Then, carefully flip the omelet and finish cooking the other side. Transfer to a warmed plate, put tomatoes and mushroom in the middle and fold.

Mediterranean Burger

Ingredients:

1/2 Cup avocado, peel & slice	1/2 Tsp. garlic powder
2 lg. leaves fresh spinach-chopped	1/2 Tbsp. parsley, chopped
1 Small tomato, sliced	1 Tbsp. onion, chopped
1 whole-wheat pita bread, toasted	1 Tbsp. extra-virgin olive oil
1/2 Cup lentils, cooked and drained	Salt & pepper to taste

Directions:

Puree lentils in processor

Place all ingredients except pita bread into a bowl and mix. Form mixture into patties. Spray pan with olive oil and heat. Place patties into pan and cook on each side for 3 min and turn. Cook another 3 min. Serve.

Salmon and Sweet Potato Puree

Ingredients:

3 Oz. salmon fish, raw	salad dressing
1 Small sweet potato, cooked (with peel)	1 tsp Smart Balance Light spread
1 Cup fresh asparagus, cooked	Garlic powder
1 Oz. feta cheese	Salt
1/2 Tbsp. homemade Italian	Pepper

Directions:

Season the salmon with salt, pepper and garlic powder. Heat olive oil spray in a non-stick pan over medium-high heat. Start salmon, with the skin faced down, cook until the fish flakes easily and is cooked through, about 3 to 4 minutes on each side. Transfer the salmon to a plate.

Meanwhile, peel the sweet potato and take to the potato masher to make a puree. Add some salt, and one teaspoon of Smart Balance. Add to plate. Season the asparagus with salad dressing and salt. Add to plate.

Serve all on a warmed plate.

Oatmeal Pancakes

Ingredients:

1/2 Cup oat flakes, raw	1 Pinch of salt
1/4 Cup milk, skimmed non-fat	1 Medium 8" banana
1/2 Beaten egg	4 chopped walnuts
Splenda	

Directions:

Place in a bowl all ingredients, except banana, and mix. Allow to rest for 10 minutes.

Heat a non-stick pan over medium heat, place two tablespoon of the mix to form pancakes and cook it until they are dry and golden.

Serve in a platter with the sliced banana and nuts.

Delicious Spaghetti

Ingredients:

1 Cup broccoli, cooked

1/3 Cup lentils, cooked

1 Cup white mushrooms, Sliced

1/2 Cup whole-wheat spaghetti, cooked

1 Cup sundried tomatoes

2 Ounce tuna in water, drained

1/2 Tbsp. extra-virgin olive oil

Salt

Pepper

Oregano

Directions:

Heat the olive oil in a wok over medium heat; add mushrooms, broccoli, tomatoes, tuna and lentils. Add salt and pepper and sauté for about 3 minutes. Add spaghetti, sauté for 2 more minutes.

Transfer to a platter and sprinkle with the oregano.

Tip:

Add the raw broccoli florets to a large pot of boiling, salted water and cook until al dente, about 3 minutes. Remove the florets and pat dry. Add the spaghetti in the same pot of water. Cook until al dente, about 8 minutes.

Chicken and Rice Marvel

Ingredients:

2 Ounce chicken breast, diced

1 Cup eggplant cubes, boiled

1/2 Cup brown long-grain rice, cooked

1Tbsp. parmesan cheese, grated

1/2 Tbsp. extra-virgin olive oil

Salt

Pepper

Directions:

Season the chicken with salt and pepper.

In a bowl, place one liter of water, add 1 tablespoon of sea salt. Wash the eggplant and remove the top and bottom ends, and cut in ½ inch slices. Put in the bowl and leave there for 2 minutes. Drain, cut in cubes, and cook in boiling water for 2 minutes and drain.

Heat the olive oil in a wok over medium heat, add chicken, stir and cook about 5 minutes, add eggplant, and stir. Add rice, stir again. Cook for 2 minutes.

Transfer to a platter; sprinkle top with the parmesan cheese.

Tip:

Cook rice: In a medium saucepan, add 1 cup of raw brown rice, 2 1/4 cold water and 1/2 tsp. of salt, and stir. Cover and allow simmering for 45 to 55 minutes.

Tuna Toast

Ingredients:

1 Whole-wheat bread slice, toasted

1 Oz. tuna in water

1/2 Cup tomato, diced

2 Basil leaves, chopped

1/2 Tbsp. extra-virgin olive oil

Salt

Pepper

Directions:

In a bowl place tuna, tomato, basil, olive oil, salt and pepper. Mix it.

 Place the toasted bread on plate. Top with this salad.

Bon Appetite.

Hummus

Ingredients:

1 cup chickpeas, cooked

1 Lemon juice

3 Tbsp. extra-virgin olive oil

1 Tbsp. Tahini

1/2 Tbsp. garlic powder

1 Tbsp. parsley, chopped

Water

Salt

Cumin Directions:

Puree chickpeas in food processor Add lemon juice, olive oil, tahini, garlic and parsley. Process again. Add some water if necessary.

Transfer to a glass container, and sprinkle with the cumin.

Minestrone

Ingredients:

2 Tbsp. extra-virgin olive oil

1 large onion, diced

2 Tbsp. garlic powder

2 stalks of celery, diced

1 large carrot, diced

1/2 Cup tomatoes, diced

1/2 Cup tomatoes, crushed

6 Cups chicken broth

1 Cup kidney beans, drained and rinsed

1 Cup whole-wheat elbow pasta

1/3 Cup parmesan cheese, grated

1 Cup green beans, trimmed and cut

1 Tsp. oregano

2 Tsp Basil

Directions:

Heat the olive oil in a large pot over medium-high heat. Add the onion and cook until translucent, about 4 minutes. Add celery, carrot and garlic and cook until they begin to soften, about 5 minutes. Add the green beans, oregano and half basil (1 tbsp.), 1/2 teaspoon salt, and pepper; cook 3 minutes.

Add the diced and crushed tomatoes and the chicken broth to the pot and bring to a boil. Reduce heat to medium low and simmer 10 minutes. Stir in kidney beans and pasta and cook until pasta and vegetables are tender, about 10 minutes. Ladle into bowls and top with the parmesan and remaining tbsp. chopped basil. Add salt & pepper to taste.

Couscous and Chicken

Ingredients:

1/2 Cup white beans, boiled

2 Ounce chicken breast, raw, diced

3/4 Cup couscous, cooked

1 Cup tomato diced

1/2 Tbsp. extra-virgin olive oil

1/2 Tsp. dried thyme

Salt, Pepper

Directions:

Heat olive oil in a medium non-stick pan over medium heat; add the chicken. Cook for 5 minutes. Add tomato, thyme and salt. Reduce the heat to minimum and cook about 10 minutes. Add the boiled white beans. Check the salt.

In the middle of a plate, place heated couscous, and around the couscous place the tomato and chicken stew.

Mediterranean Toast

Ingredients:

1 Whole-wheat bread slice, toasted	2 Basil leaves, chopped
½ Cup Tomato, diced	3 Black olives
1 Tbsp. parmesan cheese	Salt
½ Tbsp. extra-virgin olive oil	Pepper
	Oregano

Directions:

In a glass bowl place tomatoes, salt, pepper, olive oil, oregano and basil; mix it.

Place the warm toast on a plate, fill with the tomato salad. Sprinkle with cheese.

Tip:

mix cheese with bread crumbs and melted butter and slip under broiler for a few minutes

Mushroom Burger

Ingredients:

1/2 Cup sliced avocado

1 Cup white mushrooms, sliced

1 whole-wheat pita bread, toasted

1/2 Cup lentils, cooked, dried

1 Tsp. garlic powder

2 Tbsp. parsley, chopped

3 Tbsp. onion, chopped

1 Tbsp. extra-virgin olive oil

Salt

Pepper

Directions:

Using the food processor, blend the lentils until they become a paste, add ½ tbsp. of garlic powder, salt, 1 tbsp. chopped onion and 1 tbsp. parsley, and mix well. Shape into patties and cook on griddle or pan (may spray with non-stick spray) over medium heat, until nicely browned (about 6 minutes per side).

Heat the olive oil in a medium pan over medium heat, add mushrooms and stir. Add chopped onion, garlic, parsley, salt and pepper. Cook for about 5 minutes. Put aside.

Open the pita bread; place the burger inside along with avocado, mushrooms, salt and pepper.

Halibut

Ingredients:

3 Oz. fish halibut

1/2 Cup broccoli, boiled

1/2 Cauliflower, boiled

1/2 Cup brown rice, cooked

1/2 tbsp. extra-virgin olive oil

Salt

Pepper

Thyme

Directions:

Spread some olive oil on the fish, season it with thyme, salt and pepper. To broil, place the fish (the skin of the fish should be up) on the top rack of the oven and set it to broil. You can also broil it in a toaster oven. Time, about 7 minutes.

Transfer to a warmed platter.

Add the raw broccoli and cauliflowers florets to a large pot of boiling, salted water and cook until al dente, about 3 minutes. Remove the florets and pat dry.

Place on the platter along with Fish and rice. Sprinkle with a few drops of olive oil and pepper

Tip:

Cook the rice. In a medium saucepan, add 1 cup of raw brown rice, 2 1/4 cold water and 1/2 tsp. of salt, and stir. Cover and allow simmering for 45 to 55 minutes.

Mushroom Omelet

Ingredients:

1 Slice toasted whole-wheat bread

1 Tbsp. parsley, chopped

2 Eggs, beaten

1 tbsp. extra-virgin olive oil

1 Cup white mushrooms, sliced

Salt

1/2 Tbsp. garlic powder

Pepper

Directions:

Cut mushrooms into thin slices. Heat some olive oil spray in a non-stick pan over medium heat, add the mushrooms. Cook for about two minutes. Season it with salt and pepper. Meanwhile, in a small bowl beat together the eggs, add one tablespoon of cold water and season with salt and pepper.

Heat olive oil in a 20" non-stick frypan over medium heat. Add the eggs. Cook until the bottom is golden. Then, carefully flip the omelet and finish cooking the other side. Transfer to a warmed plate, place mushroom in the middle and fold.

APPENDIX A

Hummus Pita Sandwich

Ingredients:

1 Whole-wheat pita bread

2 Cup mezclum lettuce

(Arugula, endive, spinach, purslane, endive, mustard greens, beet greens, chicory)

4 Cherry Tomatoes

½ Tbsp. homemade Italian salad dressing

½ Cup hummus, commercial or homemade

Salt

Directions:

In a glass bowl place the different lettuces and tomatoes cut into quarters, season it with salt and salad dressing.

Toast the bread, open it, spread some hummus inside and fill with this colorful salad.

Bon Appetite

> **Tip:**
>
> Lettuce must be washed carefully and placed in a bowl with water and white vinegar for 5 minutes before use. Also must be cut with a plastic knife or by hand.

Vermicelli and Shrimps

Ingredients:

3 ounces raw shrimps, peeled

1/2 Cup tomato, diced

1/2 boiled zucchini, diced

1 Cup whole-wheat Vermicelli, cooked

1/2 Tbsp. extra-virgin olive oil

1 Tbsp. parmesan cheese

Salt

Pepper

Oregano

Directions:

Heat olive oil in a wok over medium heat; add shrimp and cook for 20 seconds, add tomatoes, and zucchini. Season with salt and pepper, sauté for about 3 minutes. Add spaghetti, sauté for 2 more minutes.

Transfer to a platter and sprinkle with the cheese and oregano.

Chicken and Hummus Wrap

Ingredients:

½ Cooked chicken breast, chopped

2 Tbsp. humus, commercial or homemade

1/2 Cup fresh watercress

1/2 Tsp. extra-virgin olive oil

Salt

1 Whole-wheat wrap

Directions:

Place the chicken in a bowl with watercress, a little salt and olive oil. Mix gently. You can add some red wine vinegar drops.

Heat a griddle and place the wrap. Warm it in both sides.

In a plate place the wrap, spread hummus in the surface, put some salad in the center. Wrap

Chickpeas and Tuna

Ingredients:

2/3 Cup chickpeas, cooked

3 Ounce Tuna in water

1/2 Cup cauliflower, cooked

6 Black olives

1 Tbsp. red onion, chopped

1 Tbsp. parsley, chopped

1 Tbsp. homemade Italian salad dressing

Salt

Pepper

1 whole-wheat dinner roll

Directions:

In a bowl place the chickpeas, tuna, cauliflower, olives, onion, parsley, salt, pepper, and salad dressing. Mix it carefully and serve.

Eggplant and Red Belly Pepper Salad

Ingredients:

1 Cup eggplant and red belly pepper salad

1 whole-wheat pita bread

Salad:

1 Large eggplant

1 Red belly pepper

2 Tbsp. Coriander

2 Tbsp. homemade salad dressing

1 whole-wheat pita bread

Salt/Pepper

Directions:

Place one liter of water in a bowl, add 1 tablespoon of sea salt. Remove top and bottom ends from the eggplant, and cut in ½ inch slices. Put in the bowl and leave there for 2 minutes. Cook in a non-stick grill for about 3 or 4 minutes each side or until is done. Set aside.

Place the red pepper directly on the stove fire to burn all around, until is totally black outside. Put in a plastic bag until is warm.

Wash the pepper carefully to remove all the burned skin and seeds.

Place eggplant on a cutting surface and cut into Julienne. Do the same with the pepper.

In a glass bowl, place eggplant, pepper, coriander, salt and salad dressing. Mix together